Head and Neck Cancer Clinics

Series editors
Rehan Kazi
Head and Neck Cancer
Manipal University
Manipal, India

Raghav C. Dwivedi
Head and Neck Cancer
Royal Marsden Hospital
London, United Kingdom

Head and Neck Cancer (HNC) is a major challenge to public health. Its management involves a multidisciplinary team approach, which varies depending on the subtle differences in the location of the tumour, stage and biology of disease and availability of resources. In the wake of rapidly evolving diagnostic technologies and management techniques, and advances in basic sciences related to HNC, it is important for both clinicians and basic scientists to be up-to-date in their knowledge of new diagnostic and management protocols. This series aims to cover the entire range of HNC-related issues through independent volumes on specific topics. Each volume focuses on a single topic relevant to the current practice of HNC, and contains comprehensive chapters written by experts in the field. The reviews in each volume provide vast information on key clinical advances and novel approaches to enable a better understanding of relevant aspects of HNC. Individual volumes present different perspectives and have the potential to serve as stand-alone reference guides. We believe these volumes will prove useful to the practice of head and neck surgery and oncology, and medical students, residents, clinicians and general practitioners seeking to develop their knowledge of HNC will benefit from them.

More information about this series at http://www.springer.com/series/13779

Frederick L. Greene • Andrzej L. Komorowski
Editors

Clinical Approach to Well-differentiated Thyroid Cancers

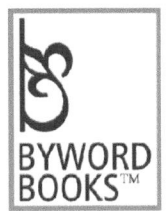

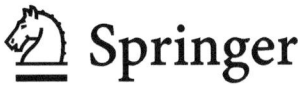

Editors
Frederick L. Greene
General Surgery
Carolinas Medical Center
Charlotte
North Carolina
USA

Andrzej L. Komorowski
General Surgery
Hospital Virgen del Camino
Sanlúcar de Barrameda
Spain

ISSN 2364-4060   ISSN 2364-4079   (electronic)
Head and Neck Cancer Clinics
ISBN 978-81-322-2567-6   ISBN 978-81-322-2568-3   (eBook)
DOI 10.1007/978-81-322-2568-3

Library of Congress Control Number: 2015953342

Springer New Delhi Heidelberg New York Dordrecht London

Cover illustration by Dan Gibbons DCR(R), PgCert(CT)

Printed on acid-free paper

Springer (India) Pvt. Ltd. is part of Science+Business Media (www.springer.com)

Dedicated to the memory of my grandfathers
Władysław Roman Bochenek, engineer, prisoner of the Gross Rosen and Mittelbau-Dora German Concentration Camps, who taught me the love for the unspoiled nature

and

Adam Ignacy Komorowski, master in goldsmithery, soldier of the Polish First Army, who taught me the meaning of the word Katyń

ALK

This series is dedicated to the research and charity efforts of Cancer Aid and Research Foundation (CARF), Mumbai, India (www.cancerarfoundation.org).

Preface

'Disease is very old and nothing about it has changed. It is we who change as we understand what was formerly imperceptible.'

—Jean Martin Charcot (1825–1893)

Differentiated thyroid cancer belongs to the small group of human malignancies with very good prognosis. Excellent outcomes result from the unique tumour biology and constantly improving treatment options. This book has been constructed as a concise clinical guide to the current management of this tumour.

The authors come from nine countries and four continents. The wide geographical distribution and different clinical background of each author result in a unique perspective on a clinical problem. As a rule, the commentaries are written by specialists based in a country other than the country of the author of the chapter.

Some topics are covered by more than one chapter; this is because we believe that each part of this book should be 'functionally' complete to avoid browsing through the pages in search of information that should logically appear also in the chapter the reader is currently reading.

We do hope that this book will help our readers to treat their patients better. We will be more than happy to receive feedback (z5komoro@cyf-kr.edu.pl). This way, the editors can also do better in the future.

Charlotte, NC, USA   Frederick L. Greene
Sanlúcar de Barrameda, Spain   Andrzej L. Komorowski

Abbreviations

AGES	Age, grade, extent, size
AJCC	American Joint Committee on Cancer
AMES	Age, metastasis, extent, size
BSRTC	Bethesda System for Reporting Thyroid Cytopathology
CLND	Central lymph node dissection
CT	Computed tomography
DTC	Differentiated thyroid carcinoma
DVT	Deep vein thrombosis
EORTC	European Organization for Research and Treatment of Cancer
ESPEN	European Society for Clinical Nutrition and Metabolism
FAP	Familial adenomatous polyposis
FDG	18-Fluoro-2-deoxyglucose
FNA	Fine needle aspirate
FNAB	Fine-needle aspiration biopsy
FNAC	Fine-needle aspiration cytology
FTC	Follicular thyroid carcinoma
GLUT	Glucose transporters
IONM	Intraoperative nerve monitoring
iPTH	Intraoperative parathyroid hormone
JCAHO	Joint Commission on Accreditation of Healthcare Organizations
MACIS	Metastases, age, completeness of resection, invasion, size
MIVAT	Minimally invasive video-assisted thyroidectomy
MRI	Magnetic resonance imaging
NCCN	National Comprehensive Cancer Network
NCDB	National Cancer Data Base
NCI	National Cancer Institute
NSCLC	Non-small cell lung cancer
PAX8-PARγ	Peroxisome proliferator-activated receptor-gamma
PEG	Percutaneous endoscopic tube
PET-CT	Positron emission tomography-CT
PTC	Papillary thyroid carcinoma
RET	Rearranged during transfection
rhTSH	Recombinant human thyroid-stimulating hormone
RLN	Recurrent laryngeal nerve

SEER	Surveillance, Epidemiology, and End Results
SPECT	Single-photon emission computerized tomography
SSI	Surgical site infection
TE	Tracheo-oesophageal
Tg	Thyroglobulin
TgAb	Thyroglobulin antibodies
TNM	Tumour–node–metastasis
TOVAT	Transoral video-assisted thyroidectomy
TSH	Thyroid-stimulating hormone
US	Ultrasound
WBS	Whole-body isotope scan
WDTC	Well-differentiated thyroid carcinoma

Contents

Contributors

Marcin Barczyński Department of Endocrine Surgery,
3rd Chair of General Surgery, Jagiellonian University, Medical College,
Krakow, Poland

Tahar Benhidjeb Department of General, Visceral and Thoracic Surgery,
University Medical Center Hamburg-Eppendorf, Hamburg, Germany

Carmine De Bartolomeis Department of Surgery, University of Pisa,
Ospedale Santa Chiara, Pisa, Italy

Istvan Gal Department of Surgery, Telki International Private Hospital,
Telki, Hungary

Frederick L. Greene Department of General Surgery, Carolinas Medical Center,
Charlotte, NC, USA

Stephen J. Gwyther Department of Radiology, East Surrey Hospital, Redhill,
Surrey, UK

Daria Handkiewicz-Junak Department of Nuclear Medicine
and Endocrine Oncology, Maria Skłodowska-Curie Memorial Cancer Center
and Institute of Oncology, Gliwice Branch, Gliwice, Poland

Pietro Iacconi Department of Surgery, University of Pisa, Ospedale Santa Chiara,
Pisa, Italy

Barbara Jarząb Department of Nuclear Medicine and Endocrine Oncology,
Maria Skłodowska-Curie Memorial Cancer Center and Institute of Oncology,
Gliwice Branch, Gliwice, Poland

R. Kalyani Department of Pathology, Sri Devaraj Urs Medical College,
Sri Devaraj Urs Academy of Higher Education and Research, Sri R.L. Jalappa
Hospital and Research Centre, Kolar, Karnataka, India

Stanislaw Kłęk Department of General Surgery, 1st Chair of General Surgery,
Jagiellonian University Medical College and Nutrimed Medical Corporation,
Krakow, Poland

Andrzej L. Komorowski Department of General Surgery, Hospital Virgen del Camino, Sanlúcar de Barrameda, Spain

Artur Komorowski Department of Medical Education, Jagiellonian University, Medical College, Krakow, Poland

Department of Radiology, Maria Skłodowska-Curie Memorial Cancer Center and Institute of Oncology, Krakow, Poland

Markus Luster Department of Nuclear Medicine, University of Ulm, Ulm, Germany

Gabriele Materazzi Department of Surgery, University of Pisa, Pisa, Italy

Ettienne J. Myburgh Department of Surgery, Panorama Medi-Clinic and Head, Neck and Breast Unit, Tygerberg Academic Hospital, Cape Town, South Africa

Josephine N. Rini Department of Nuclear Medicine, Albert Einstein College of Medicine of Yeshiva University, Bronx, NY, USA

North Shore-LIJ Center for Advanced Medicine, New Hyde Park, NY, USA

Mitchell Goldman Diagnostic Imaging Center, Lake Success, New York, USA

Janusz Ryś Department of Tumour Pathology, Maria Skłodowska-Curie Memorial Cancer Center and Institute of Oncology, Krakow, Poland

Amit Vats Department of Biosurgery and Surgical Technology, Imperial College, St Mary's Hospital, London, UK

Joanna Wysocka Department of Tumour Pathology, Maria Skłodowska-Curie Memorial Cancer Center and Institute of Oncology, Krakow, Poland

Andrzej M. Wysocki Department of General Surgery, 2nd Chair of General Surgery, Jagiellonian University, Medical College, Krakow, Poland

Wojciech M. Wysocki Department of Surgical Oncology, Maria Skłodowska-Curie Memorial Cancer Center and Institute of Oncology, Krakow, Poland

Historical Perspective and Current Epidemiology

Wojciech M. Wysocki and Andrzej L. Komorowski

In this chapter we present a brief history of the treatment of thyroid cancer and its current epidemiology.

History

The most visible sign of thyroid pathology is goitre (Fig. 1.1), and for centuries it was referred to as bronchocoele ('tracheal out-pouch'). As the gland itself resembles the shield commonly used in ancient Greece, the term thyroid – meaning shield – was coined in 1656 by Thomas Wharton. The 'shield' core is reflected in the gland's name in many languages (German *schilddrüse* [schild=shield], Polish *tarczyca* [tarcza=shield]).

The pathophysiology of the thyroid gland was unclear to physicians for a relatively long time. Iodine was discovered in 1811 by Bernard Courtois while isolating sodium and potassium from seaweed ash; 2 years later William Prout used iodine to treat thyroid goitre for the first time. Robert James Graves, in 1835, gave the first complete description of exophthalmic goitre.

In 1833, goitre was first differentiated from thyroid cancer by Allan Burns and Gaspard Bayle. Thyroiditis, as a clinical entity distinct from goitre, was described by Bernhard Riedel in 1896.

The first reported resection of the thyroid gland was made by Pierre Joseph Dasault in 1796. However, thyroid surgery was at that time considered extremely dangerous because of massive haemorrhages, multiple complications and high

W.M. Wysocki
Department of Surgical Oncology, Maria Skłodowska-Curie Memorial Cancer Center and Institute of Oncology, Krakow, Poland

A.L. Komorowski (✉)
Department of General Surgery, Hospital Virgen del Camino, Sanlúcar de Barrameda, Spain
e-mail: z5komoro@cyf-kr.edu.pl

© The Author(s) 2012
F.L. Greene, A.L. Komorowski (eds.), *Clinical Approach to Well-differentiated Thyroid Cancers*, Head and Neck Cancer Clinics,
DOI 10.1007/978-81-322-2568-3_1

Fig. 1.1 A man with a large goitre. Coloured engraving from Alexandre Auvert's *Selecta Praxis Medico-Chirurgicae quam Mosquae exercet alexander Auvert,* Paris, 1851 (Courtesy of Professor Amelio Dolfi, Biblioteca di Medicina e Chirurgia dell'Università di Pisa)

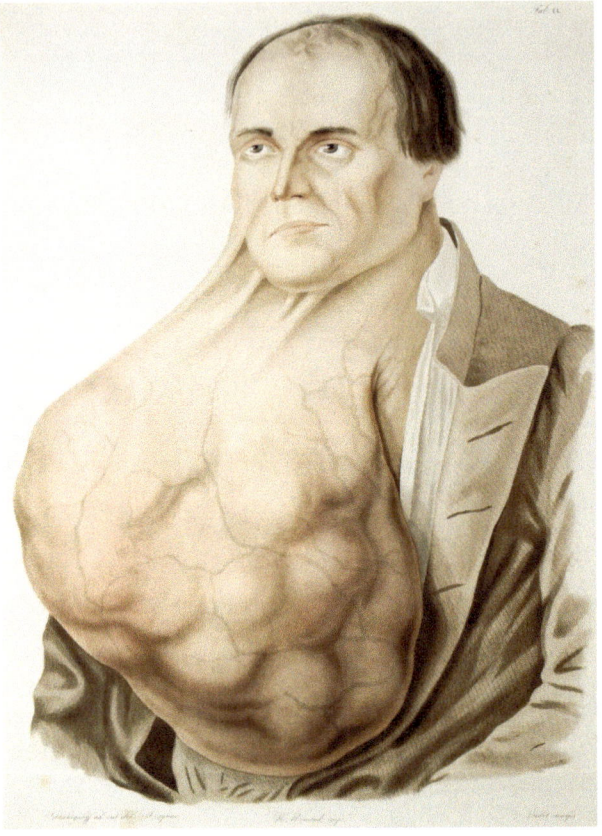

mortality. Many surgeons declared themselves as determined opponents of surgical treatment of thyroid gland diseases. Proponents of thyroid surgery, like Luigi Porta, proposed to divide the thyroid arteries in order to cut off the blood supply to the thyroid. It was not until the end of the 19th century that surgeons started operating on the thyroid with acceptable results, with the aid of anaesthesia and antiseptics. The first total thyroidectomy was performed in 1880 by Ludwig Rehn. Five years later Jan Mikulicz-Radecki performed the first subtotal thyroidectomy. The surgical treatment of the thyroid gland was developed quicker in areas with endemic goitre, such as Switzerland. Theodor Kocher, a surgeon from Berne, extensively studied thyroid gland physiology and developed modern techniques for thyroid surgery. He was awarded the Nobel Prize in medicine in 1909 for his studies on thyroid hormones. In subsequent years, surgery of the thyroid gland has become increasingly widespread (Fig. 1.2). Charles Horace Mayo and his co-worker, Henry Plummer, made important progress in the field of pathophysiology and surgery of the thyroid gland, as did William Stewart Halsted. In 1912, a bioactive substance from the thyroid gland was isolated by Edward Kendall (Nobel

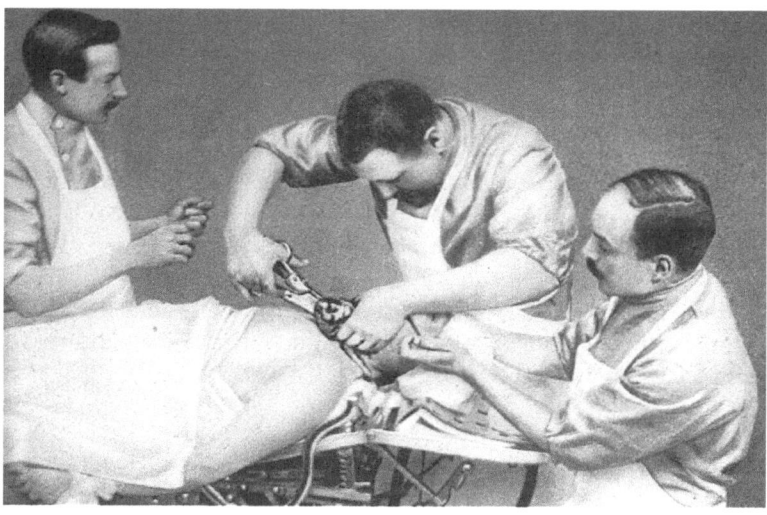

Fig. 1.2 French surgeon Eugène Doyen from Paris performing thyroidectomy in 1914 (Image property Bibliothèque de l'Académie Nationale de Médecine, with permission)

Prize laureate in 1950) and named thyroxin. The discovery of radioactive iodine isotope by Frederic and Irene Joliot-Curie in 1934 started a new era in the diagnosis and treatment of thyroid diseases.

Epidemiology

Thyroid malignancies presently account for 1–1.5 % of all malignancies in men. This group of diseases is the most common among all endocrine malignancies (thyroid malignancies account for 90 % of all endocrine malignancies).

Differentiated thyroid carcinomas constitute ~95 % of thyroid malignancies. There are three major types of differentiated carcinomas (papillary, follicular, Hürthle-cell), which represent 60–90 % of all differentiated cancers. The most commonly encountered differentiated thyroid carcinoma is papillary (60–80 %), followed by follicular (10–20 %) and Hürtle-cell type (2–5 %). Production and secretion of thyroglobulin is a specific feature of all types of differentiated thyroid cancers.

The disease develops mainly in women (~70 %). The male-to-female ratio depends on the age at diagnosis; the incidence in men and women is almost equal in childhood and in the elderly, but female predominance is noted in the early and middle adult years (this is perhaps related to the expression of oestrogen receptors on neoplastic thyroid epithelium). The standardized incidence varies greatly worldwide: 0.8–5/100,000/year in men and 1.9–19.4/100,000/year in women. The incidence of thyroid cancer increased almost 310 % between 1950 and 2004. Such an increase in the incidence could be explained by the addition of iodine to common food products, a change in pathological criteria for the diagnosis of thyroid cancer, and common use of imaging modalities resulting in the rise of the number of incidental thyroid cancers, i.e. cancers found by coincidence without clinical symptoms. Despite the growing incidence, the mortality from this disease decreased, i.e. by almost 45 % from 1950 to 1975, and remained stable or slowly decreased thereafter. This decrease is due to improved diagnosis and treatment modalities as well as the indolent nature of differentiated thyroid cancers. The 10-year relative survival rates for papillary, follicular and Hürthle-cell thyroid cancers were 95 %, 83 % and 76 %, respectively. Despite the fact that differentiated thyroid cancers develop two to three times more frequently in women, the majority of deaths from this disease occur in male patients, as men are usually diagnosed at a more advanced age and more advanced stage of the disease.

Suggested Reading

Amos KD, Habra MA, Perrier ND. Carcinoma of the thyroid and parathyroid glands. In: Feig BW, Berger DH and Fuhrman GM (eds). *The MD Anderson surgical oncology handbook*. Philadelphia; 2006.
Brucer M. Nuclear medicine begins with a boa constrictor. *J Nucl Med* 1978;**19**:581–98.
Fragu P. Le regard de l'histoire des sciences sûr la glande thyroïde (1800–1960). *Ann Endocrinol (Paris)* 1999;**60**:10–22.

Pathology of Differentiated Thyroid Cancers

2

Janusz Ryś and Joanna Wysocka

This chapter discusses briefly the pathological aspects of differentiated thyroid cancers. The authors explain the histological features of thyroid cancers and possible approaches for making a firm diagnosis. The prognosis of different subtypes of differentiated thyroid cancer is also discussed.

Introduction

Thyroid cancers represent a heterogeneous group of neoplasms that comprise ~1 % of all human malignancies. They constitute the bulk of cancers of the endocrine system and are responsible for the majority of deaths associated with malignant endocrine neoplasms. On the basis of their morphology, clinical features and molecular characteristics of the tumour cells, these tumours have traditionally been divided into major categories of well-differentiated (papillary or follicular), medullary, and undifferentiated carcinomas. Almost 90 % of all thyroid malignancies are well-differentiated carcinomas (WDTC) that originate from the follicular epithelial cells and possess the ability to produce and release thyroid hormones. This category includes both papillary and follicular carcinomas. According to the WHO classification, the Hürthle-cell carcinoma is recognized as a variant of follicular carcinoma.

Most of the WDTCs behave like indolent tumours and have an excellent prognosis; the 5-year survival rate of patients exceeds 90 %.

J. Ryś • J. Wysocka (✉)
Department of Tumour Pathology, Maria Skłodowska-Curie Memorial Cancer Center and Institute of Oncology, Krakow, Poland
e-mail: jwysocka@mp.pl

© The Author(s) 2012
F.L. Greene, A.L. Komorowski (eds.), *Clinical Approach to Well-differentiated Thyroid Cancers*, Head and Neck Cancer Clinics,
DOI 10.1007/978-81-322-2568-3_2

Fine-Needle Aspiration Cytology of Thyroid Nodule

Fine-needle aspiration biopsy (FNAB) is a basic, common test that is considered the method of choice for diagnosis in the current recommendations for management of thyroid nodules. It is a minimally invasive procedure with enough sensitivity and specificity, which protects as many as 75 % of patients with clinically solitary nodules, thereby eliminating the need for further tests and unnecessary surgical treatment.

To minimize any disparity in diagnoses by cytopathologists/pathologists and clinicians, the Bethesda System for Reporting Thyroid Cytopathology (BSRTC) recommends that each thyroid FNAB report should begin with a general diagnostic category. The six BSRTC diagnostic categories are depicted in Table 2.1. Adequate smears are divided into four groups: (i) benign, (ii) undetermined, (iii) suspicious (groups IV–V, Table 2.1), and (iv) malignant. The benign category includes a normal thyroid, nodular

Table 2.1 The Bethesda system for reporting thyroid cytopathology; recommended diagnostic categories and risk of malignancy (according to SZ Ali and ES Cibas—modified)

Diagnostic categories of FNA of thyroid gland		Risk of malignancy (%)
I.	Non-diagnostic or unsatisfactory	
II.	Benign	0–3
	Consistent with a benign follicular nodule (includes adenomatoid nodule, colloid nodule, etc.)	
	Consistent with lymphocytic (Hashimoto) thyroiditis in the proper clinical context	
	Consistent with granulomatous (subacute) thyroiditis	
	Others	
III.	Atypia of undetermined significance or follicular lesion of undetermined significance	5–15
IV.	Follicular neoplasm or suspicious for a follicular neoplasm	15–30
	Specifying of oncocytic type of neoplasm is recommended	
V.	Suspicious for malignancy	60–75
	Suspicious for papillary carcinoma	
	Suspicious for medullary carcinoma	
	Suspicious for metastatic carcinoma	
	Suspicious for lymphoma	
VI.	Malignant	97–99
	Papillary thyroid carcinoma	
	Poorly differentiated carcinoma	
	Medullary thyroid carcinoma	
	Undifferentiated (anaplastic) carcinoma	
	Squamous cell carcinoma	
	Carcinoma with mixed features	
	Metastatic carcinoma	
	Non-Hodgkin lymphoma	

FNA fine-needle aspiration

goitre or hyperplastic/adenomatoid nodule, as well as lymphocytic or granulomatous thyroiditis. The group of malignant smears includes papillary carcinoma, medullary carcinoma, poorly differentiated and undifferentiated carcinoma, lymphoma, and met-astatic or secondary malignant neoplasm. The suspicious category concerns mainly follicular neoplasms because the cytological features of follicular carcinoma and fol-licular adenoma are undistinguishable. It also refers to oncocytic tumours (which are included in the group of follicular neoplasms). This category applies also to smears of papillary and medullary carcinomas and/or lymphomas, which lack the specific cyto-logical features required for diagnosing a malignant lesion.

In the case of thyroid cancer, the sensitivity and specificity of FNAB ranges from 65 to 98 % and from 72 to 100 %, respectively. The rate of false-negative results is estimated to vary from 1 to 11 % and the false-positive results from 0 to 7 %.

Cytological Features That Are Diagnostic of Papillary Thyroid Carcinoma

Papillary thyroid carcinoma (PTC) presents characteristic cytological features that can be recognized easily in aspirates. Typical aspirates from PTC contain an abun-dance of cells that may be grouped in three-dimensional clusters (Fig. 2.1) and syncytial-like flat sheets ('monolayers') or formed papillary arrangements. Crowding, overlapping and molding of the cancer cells are important features that distinguish them from benign follicular cells (Figs. 2.2 and 2.3). However, the

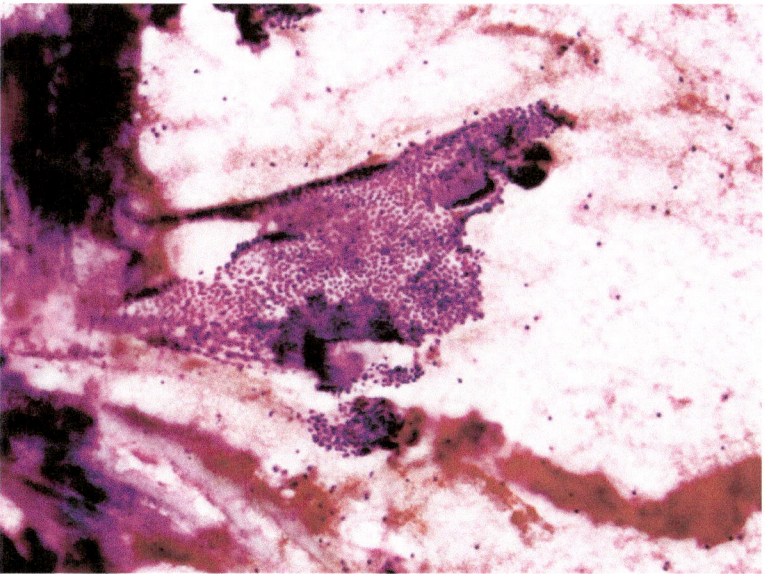

Fig. 2.1 Papillary thyroid carcinoma. Three-dimensional clusters of neoplastic cells (smear, HE stain)

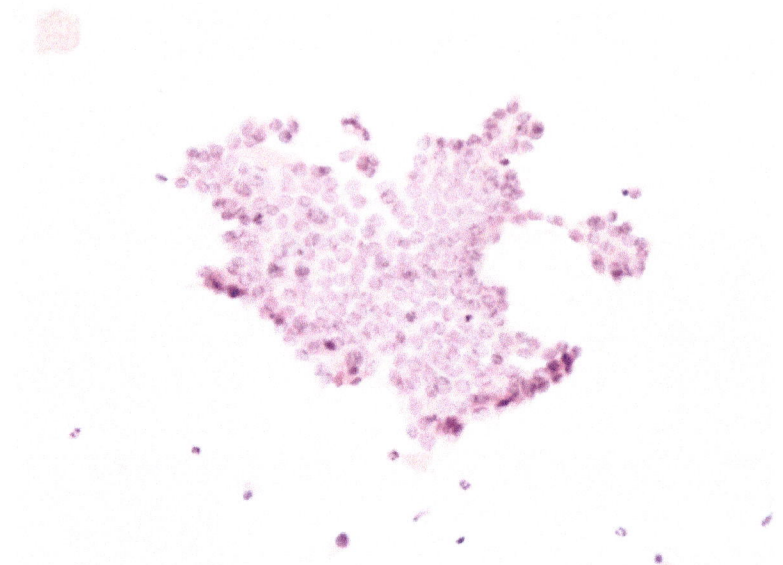

Fig. 2.2 Papillary thyroid carcinoma. Monolayer sheet of neoplastic cells with syncytial-like appearance. Notice the clearing of nuclear chromatin as well as crowding, overlapping, and molding of the cancer cells typical for papillary carcinoma (smear, HE stain)

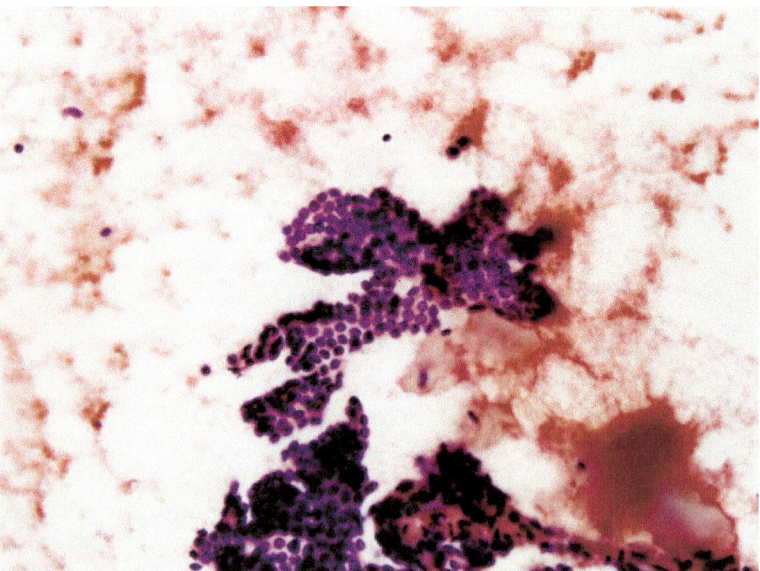

Fig. 2.3 Papillary thyroid carcinoma. Papillary-like arrangements of cancer cells (smear, HE stain)

Table 2.2 Principal nuclear features of papillary carcinoma	1. Nuclear enlargement
	2. Nuclear crowding and overlapping
	3. Chromatin clearing
	4. Irregularity of nuclear contours
	5. Intranuclear pseudoinclusions
	6. Intranuclear grooves

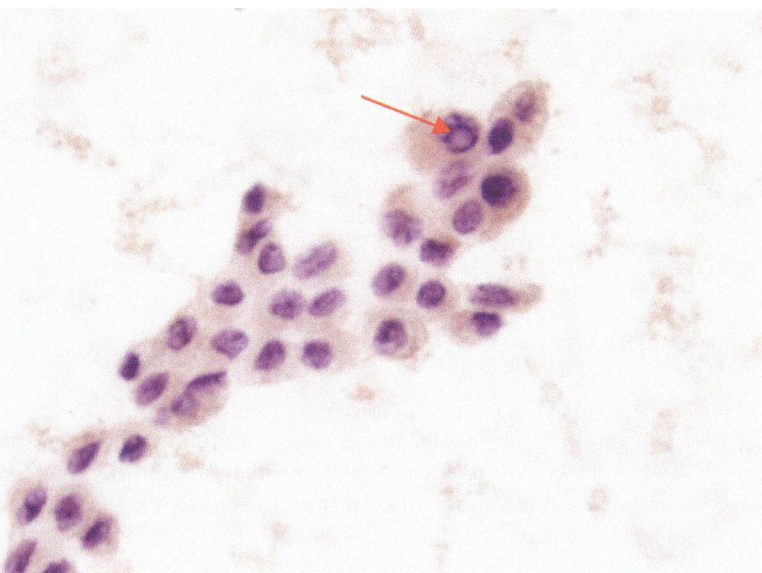

Fig. 2.4 Papillary thyroid carcinoma. Intranuclear pseudoinclusion (*red arrow*) (smear, HE stain)

defining and diagnostic features of PTC are seen in the nuclei of the cancer cells. They are typically enlarged and contain dusty-to-powdery chromatin (so-called 'ground-glass nuclei'). Furthermore, the nuclear membrane has characteristic irregularities that look like intranuclear pseudoinclusions and grooves (Table 2.2 and Figs. 2.4 and 2.5). Other typical features of PTC are multinucleated cells and bodies (rounded and lamellated calcifications). Additionally, specimens also contain droplets of ropy (or 'chewing gum') colloid.

In selected cases, the cytological picture of PTC may be confused with aspirates from papillary structures of Grave disease or papillary hyperplastic nodules. The differential diagnosis must also include hyalinized trabecular adenoma—the rare tumour of follicular cell origin characterized by trabecular growth, marked hyalinization and nuclear changes imitating completely those of PTC (nuclear inclusions and grooves, psammoma bodies).

Cytological aspirates from the follicular variant of PTC may be sometimes confused with smears from follicular neoplasms. This is because some features may be

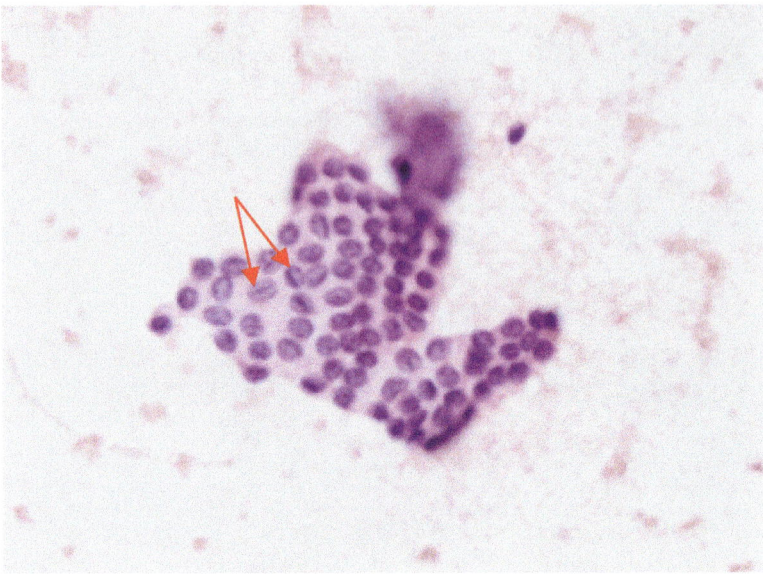

Fig. 2.5 Papillary thyroid carcinoma. The nuclear grooves (*red arrows*) (smear, HE stain)

absent, such as papillary arrangements of cells, multinucleated giant cells and psammoma bodies. Instead of papillary structures, the tumour cells form syncytial-like sheets and dispersed multifollicular clusters. However, the nuclear features of the cancer cells are typical of PTC.

Cytological Characteristics of Follicular Thyroid Carcinoma

Contrary to PTC, cytological diagnosis of follicular thyroid carcinoma (FTC) is more difficult or even impossible because of microscopic similarities in aspirates from FTC and adenoma. Smears of both FTC and follicular adenoma usually contain numerous clusters of glandular cells, often arranged in ring-like (follicular) or rosette-like acinar structures (Figs. 2.6, 2.7 and 2.8). Some of them contain inspissated colloid. Single follicular cells and nuclei stripped of cytoplasm are also visible. The presence of nuclear atypia does not reflect the malignant behaviour of tumours. Hence, the diagnosis of malignancy of a follicular tumour depends on the histological features of the neoplasm—capsular and/or vascular invasion (*see* section "Follicular carcinoma"). It is for this reason that the cytological diagnosis of 'follicular neoplasm' requires an obligatory surgical excision and microscopic examination of the tumour.

In the case of oncocytic thyroid tumours (Hürthle-cell lesions), the cytological analysis of smears also does not distinguish benign from malignant lesions. For a definitive diagnosis, a histological examination is required that can demonstrate capsular and/or vascular invasion. The cytological features of oncocytic tumours are

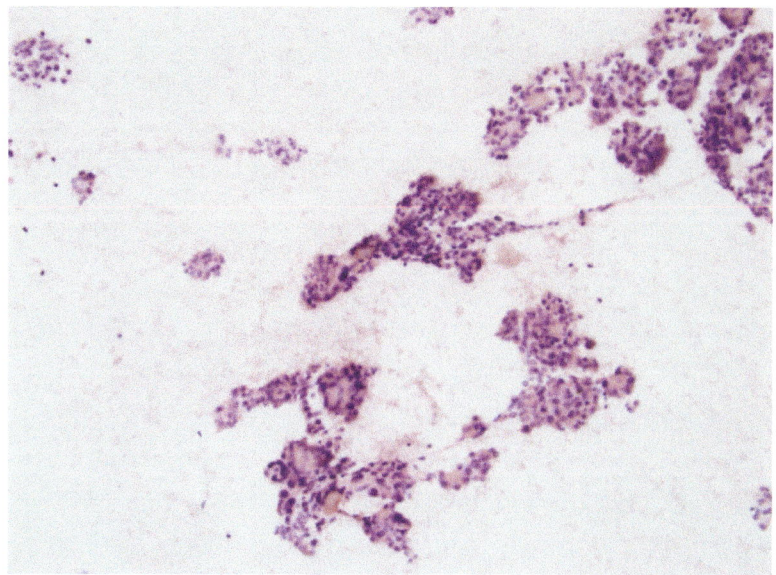

Fig. 2.6 Follicular thyroid neoplasm. Numerous clusters of glandular cells (smear, HE stain)

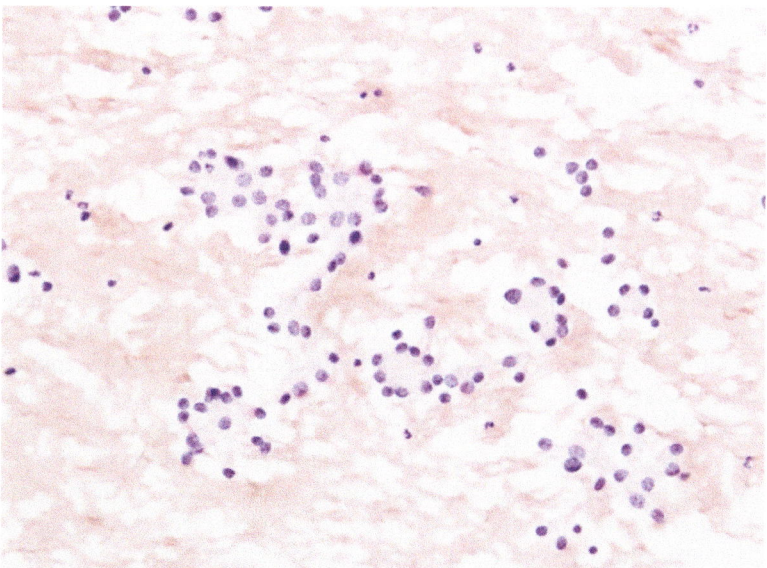

Fig. 2.7 Follicular thyroid neoplasm. Glandular cells arranged in ring-like (follicular) structures (smear, HE stain)

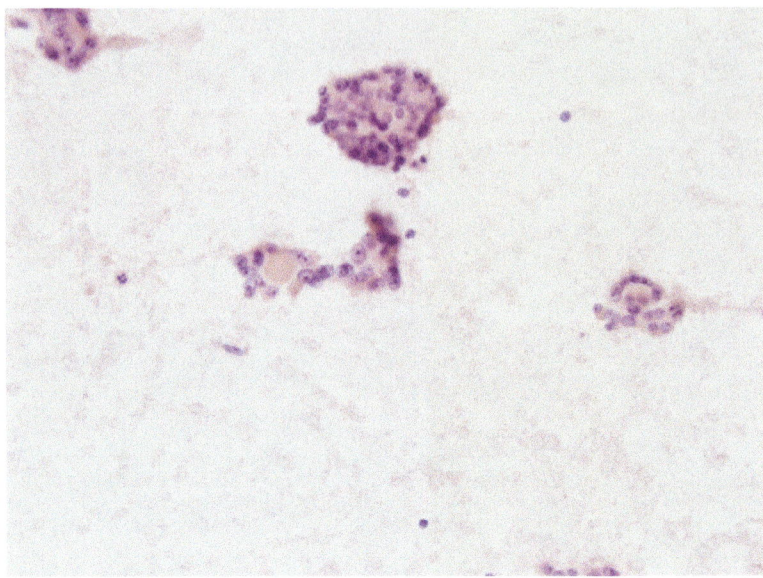

Fig. 2.8 Follicular thyroid neoplasm. Glandular cells arranged in ring-like (follicular) structures. Some of them contain inspissated colloid (smear, HE stain)

similar to those of follicular neoplasms. However, Hürthle cells are characterized by deeply eosinophilic and granular cytoplasm, and round, large, hyperchromatic nuclei with prominent nucleoli.

Why Not a Frozen Section?

The frozen section procedure is a popular and very important diagnostic method in oncological surgery; it often decreases the extent of the surgery and establishes an initial morphological diagnosis ('benign tumour' versus 'malignant tumour') during the operation. However, in the context of thyroid surgery, a practical application of this method is very limited. First, so-called 'freezing artefacts' are seen in the slides. These artificial changes in the microscopic appearance of the cells make the assessment of nuclear features impossible. Essentially, it hinders the diagnosis of PTC. Although this limitation can be excluded by the use of touch imprints (cytological preparations taken directly from the fresh specimen), the diagnostic (cytological) criteria employed here are the same as those for FNAB.

The second important issue is difficulties in differentiating between benign and malignant follicular neoplasms, as well as Hürthle-cell lesions. In these cases, a diagnosis of malignancy depends mainly on the findings of capsular and/or vascular invasion. It requires evaluation of the whole tumour capsule with extensive sampling of the specimen, which is impossible with the frozen section procedure. This limitation often is called a 'sampling error' because it is associated with an inadequate number of slices available during this rapid pathological examination.

To summarize, most authors do not recommend the use of the frozen section procedure during thyroid surgery.

Histopathology of Well-Differentiated Thyroid Carcinomas

Papillary Carcinoma

Papillary thyroid carcinoma (PTC) accounts for 80–85 % of all cases of malignant epithelial tumours of the thyroid. Most PTCs occur in adults (20–50 years of age), especially among women (female-to-male ratio 4:1). PTC also represents the most common paediatric malignancy of the thyroid gland. Multifocality is a frequent finding in these neoplasms; this phenomenon may be associated with intraglandular metastases but data from studies of the clonal rearrangements or X chromosome inactivation patterns support somewhat the simultaneous growth of multiple primary tumours in most patients.

Pathogenesis
Various environmental, hormonal and genetic factors play a role in the development of PTC. The link to radiation of the thyroid gland (derived from either external or internal sources, e.g. exposure to radioactive iodine) is well documented. The carcinogenic effect of radiation is seen particularly in young children. A clear increase in the incidence of thyroid cancer in children has been noted in Belarus after the Chernobyl disaster in 1986 (100-fold higher compared with the worldwide incidence). PTC is also considered to be associated with substantial dietary iodine intake. This type of thyroid carcinoma is three times more common in women compared to men, which suggests a hormonal influence on the pathogenesis of PTC. The rearrangements of the *RET* gene, leading to the formation of various types of *RET/PTC* oncogenes, is believed to be specific to PTC. The second most popular genetic change in PTC is point mutations of the *BRAF* and *RAS* genes.

Gross Examination
PTCs present a variety of macroscopic patterns. However, most of them are grey–white masses with irregular or sharply circumscribed margins. Sometimes, calcifications can be noticed on gross examination within the tumours. PTC can present as a solid and/or cystic tumour; entirely cystic papillary carcinomas are rare. The size of the tumour ranges from a tiny nodule (<1 mm) to a mass that is several centimetres in diameter. PTC can even involve the whole lobe of the thyroid gland and infiltrate into fat, skeletal muscle and adjacent organs (oesophagus, larynx and trachea). On the contrary, when the carcinoma's dimension is <1 cm in diameter, it is called a 'papillary microcarcinoma' (*see* later part of this section).

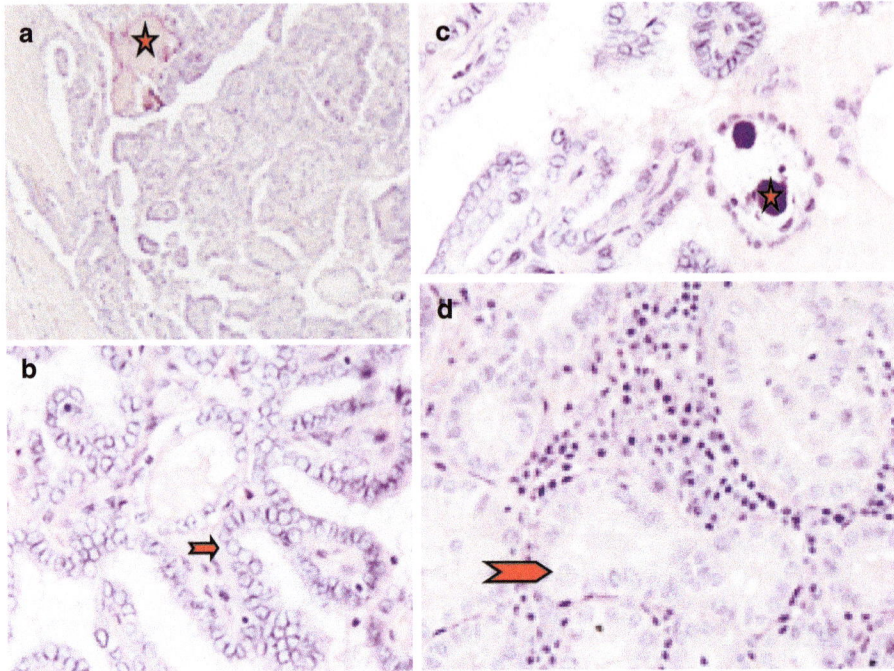

Fig. 2.9 Papillary thyroid carcinoma. (**a**–**c**) Classic type with the branching papillae covered by cells with characteristic 'ground glass' nuclei (*red arrow* on **c**) and microcalcifications (*asterisks*). (**d**) Follicular variant built of ring-like structures. The diagnosis is based on nuclear features of the cancer cell. Notice nuclear pseudoinclusion (*red arrow*) typical for papillary carcinoma (histological slide, HE stain)

Microscopic Examination

The WHO classification of thyroid tumours specifies 16 histological types of PTC (including classic/conventional variants) (Fig. 2.9). The histological division is based on the growth pattern, cytological features of tumour cells, and the type of tumour stroma. All papillary carcinomas present with the typical nuclear features (Table 2.2) that are required for diagnosing PTC. Histological subtypes of PTC are listed in Table 2.3; they differ either morphologically or clinically. Some of them may have an aggressive clinical course.

The most frequent type of PTC is the classic variant, which presents a typical papillary architecture. The papillae consist of a fibrovascular core and usually demonstrate complex branching (Figs. 2.10 and 2.11). Apart from the papillary structures, psammoma bodies and multinucleated cells can be observed.

A special variant of PTC, which requires a separate description because of its clinical importance, is a papillary microcarcinoma. This term is reserved for an incidentally found neoplasm measuring ≤10 mm in diameter. Typically, this type of PTC is characterized by a benign clinical course; however, in children it can behave more aggressively.

Table 2.3 Histological variants of papillary thyroid carcinoma (PTC) and their different prognoses (Note the types with an unfavourable prognosis)

Variants of PTC	Prognosis
Classic	Good
Follicular[a]	Similar to classic type
Good ['Similar = Good']	
Macrofollicular	Similar to other follicular variants, with lymph node metastases present in ~20 % and distant metastases in 7 % of cases
Oncocytic	Not known
Clear cell	Not known
Diffuse sclerosing	Similar to classic type (despite high incidence of regional lymph node and distant metastases)
Tall cell	Poor
Columnar cell	Poor
Solid	Poor[b]
Cribriform	Not known (usually associated with FAP [Gardner syndrome])
With fasciitis-like stroma	Similar to classic type
With focal insular component	Not known
With squamous cell or mucoepidermoid carcinoma	Poor
With spindle and giant cell carcinoma	Not known
Combined papillary and medullary carcinoma	Not known
Papillary microcarcinoma	Good (but in ≤11 % cases lymph node metastasis can be present)

[a]It is a special variant of PTC built exclusively or predominantly of follicular growth patterns. The differential diagnosis from follicular carcinoma is based on the typical nuclear features of follicular PTC, which are similar to those observed in a classical variant of papillary carcinoma
[b]Although some studies have revealed a slightly higher recurrence and mortality associated with the solid variant, most reports have shown a prognosis similar to that of classic papillary carcinoma. *FAP* familial adenomatous polyposis

Irrespective of the size of the tumour, ≤11 % of papillary microcarcinomas can be lymph node positive (according to other authors this rate is even higher and reaches 14–44 %). Ito and Miyauchi distinguish the selected clinico-morphological (high-risk) features of papillary microcarcinoma, which identify patients who need immediate surgical treatment. These features include the following: tumours located near the trachea or on the dorsal surface of the thyroid (these carcinomas show dorsal extension and invade the adjacent organs), features of a high-grade tumour in cytological material (from an FNAB), presence of regional lymph node or distant metastasis, increase in the size of tumour, and/or appearance of node metastasis. Patients with such tumours should undergo surgery.

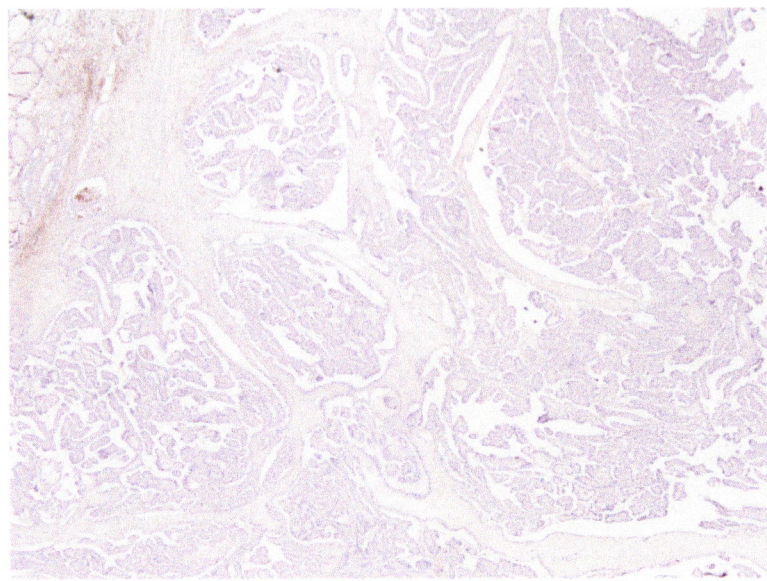

Fig. 2.10 Papillary thyroid carcinoma. Classic type with typical papillary arrangements (histological slide, HE stain)

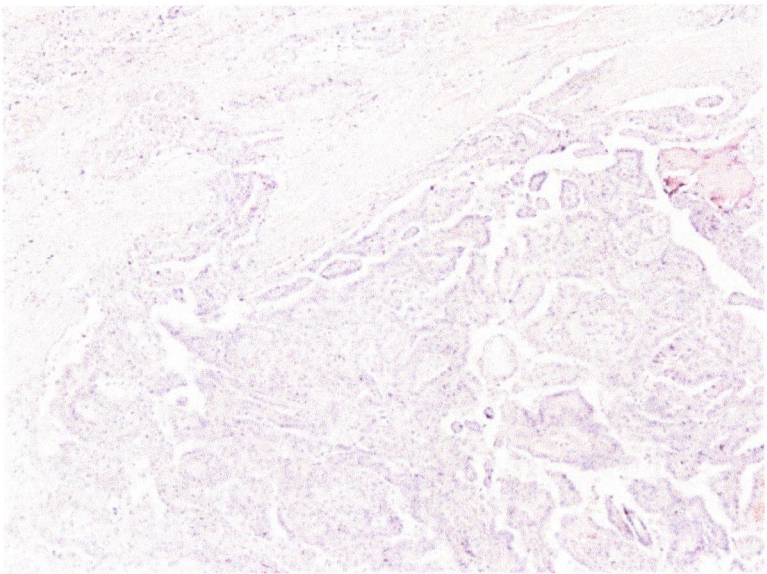

Fig. 2.11 Papillary thyroid carcinoma. Classic type with typical papillary arrangements (histological slide, HE stain)

Prognosis
Most PTCs are characterized by an excellent prognosis—the 10-year survival rate is >90 %; in the case of young patients it can even be >98 %.

Follicular Carcinoma

By definition it is a malignant epithelial tumour which shows a follicular differentiation (follicle formation) and lack of the characteristic nuclear features of papillary carcinoma. FTC accounts for 10–15 % of thyroid malignancies. It is more common in women and usually occurs in patients who are older than those with PTC. This kind of neoplasm has a much lower frequency of lymph node metastasis compared with PTC (<5 %), but distant metastases (mainly to the lung and bone) are more often present at the time of diagnosis (from 20 to 33 %, according to different authors).

Pathogenesis
Environmental and genetic factors affect the development of FTC, which is associated with dietary iodine deficiency. In this type of tumour, *RAS* mutations and *PAX8-PPAR*γ (peroxisome proliferator-activated receptor-gamma) rearrangement often can be observed.

Gross Examination
Usually follicular carcinomas are encapsulated solid tumours and their size is >1 cm. The colour of the neoplasm on cross-section varies from grey–tan to brown. In the case of widely invasive tumours, involvement of the tumour capsule can be easily seen or the capsule is altogether absent, whereas the appearance of minimally invasive carcinomas is practically identical with this type of follicular adenoma.

Microscopic Examination
The morphology of FTC is variable and includes tumours with follicles filled with colloid, and neoplasms that have solid and trabecular growth patterns (Fig. 2.12). However, the criteria for malignancy depend on the presence of vascular and/or capsular invasion; features of tumours, such as architecture or cytological atypia, are not essential for diagnosis. Generally, FTC is divided into two main groups according to the extent of tumour invasiveness—minimally invasive (with limited infiltration of the tumour capsule or through the tumour capsule and/or vascular invasion [Fig. 2.13]); and widely invasive follicular carcinoma (Fig. 2.14). The latter category includes carcinoma with distinct and wide infiltration of thyroid tissue and/or blood vessels (Table 2.4). Because of the many opinions regarding this issue, the WHO classification has defined the term 'capsular invasion' and 'vascular invasion'. A 'capsular invasion' should be recognized only when tumour cells penetrate through the capsule and this cannot be linked with the site of a previous FNAB. 'Vascular invasion' means the presence of intravascular tumour cells covered by endothelium or associated with a thrombus; it refers only to the vessels within or

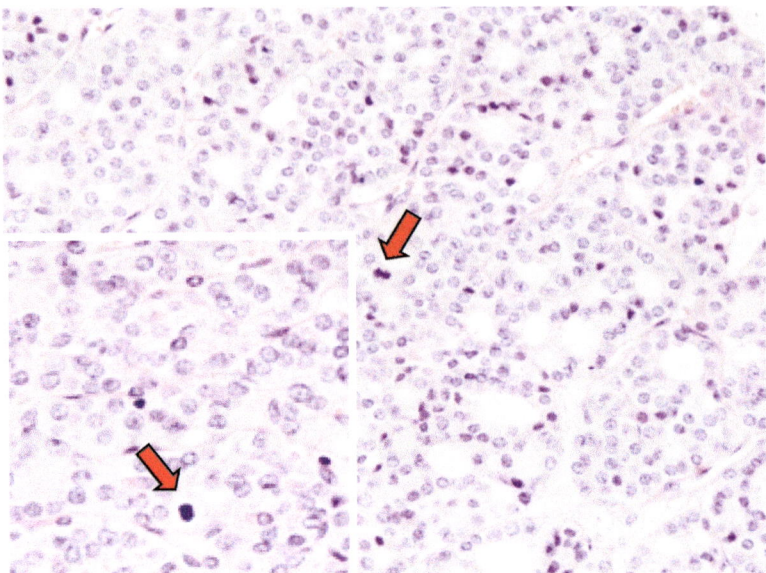

Fig. 2.12 Follicular thyroid carcinoma. Neoplastic glandular cells forming the follicles filled with colloid or the solid and trabecular patterns. Numerous mitotic figures (*red arrows*) (histological slide, HE stain)

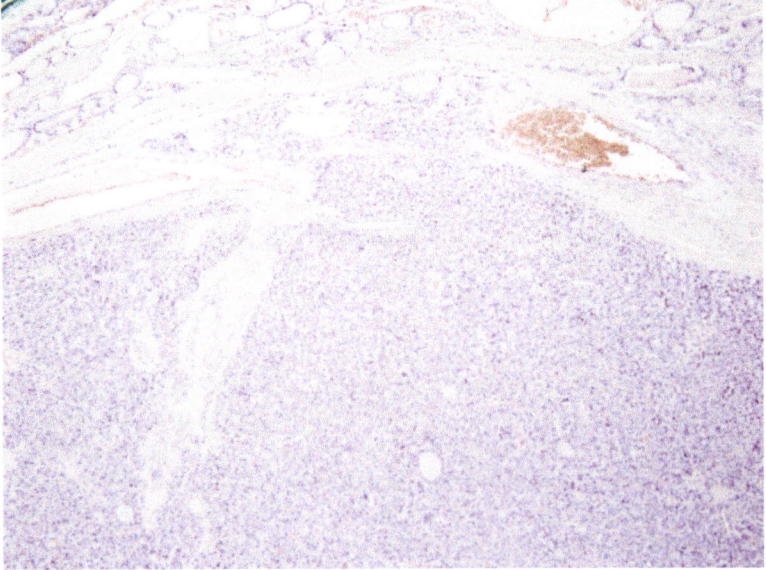

Fig. 2.13 Minimally invasive follicular thyroid carcinoma. Notice the infiltration of normal thyroid tissue outside the tumour capsule (histological slide, HE stain)

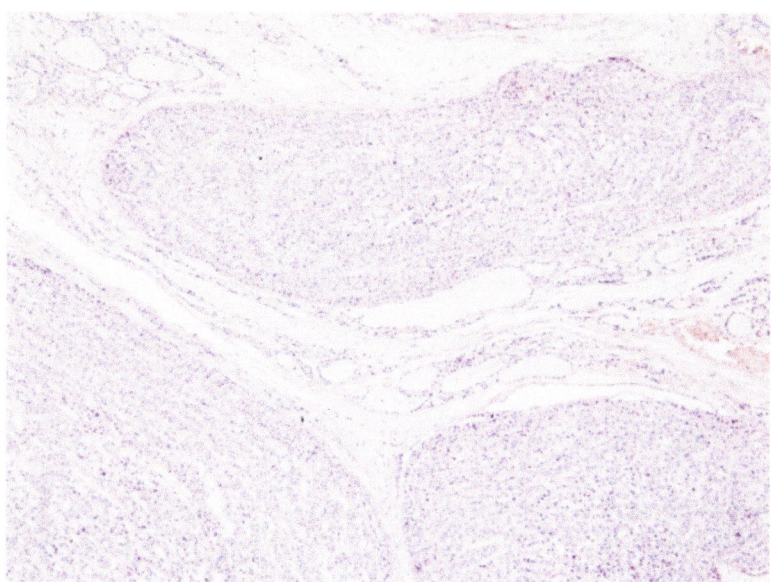

Fig. 2.14 Widely invasive follicular thyroid carcinoma. Distinct and wide infiltration of thyroid tissue (histological slide, HE stain)

Table 2.4 Histological variants of follicular thyroid carcinoma (FTC) and their different prognoses. Note the types with an unfavourable prognosis (based on Nikiforov et al.)

Variants of follicular carcinoma	Prognosis
Encapsulated FTC with microscopic capsular invasion (no vascular invasion is present) = minimally invasive follicular carcinoma	Very low probability (<5 % of cases) of metastases, recurrence or tumour-associated mortality
Encapsulated FTC with angioinvasion (capsular invasion is present or absent)	Metastases, recurrences or tumour-associated mortality in 5–30 % of cases
Widely invasive follicular carcinoma	Metastases, recurrences or tumour associated mortality in 50–55 % of cases
Oncocytic	Nodal metastases in approximately 30 % of cases
Clear cell	Not known
Mucinous variant	Not known
FTC with signet-ring cells	Not known

beyond the capsule. Some authors also use the term 'grossly encapsulated angio-invasive follicular carcinoma' to describe a tumour in which both capsular and vascular invasion is present (as opposed to minimally invasive carcinoma with only capsular invasion).

The important issue is differentiation between minimally invasive FTC and follicular adenoma and nodular goitre. Therefore, a diagnosis of this type of carcinoma can be made only after a thorough microscopic examination of the tumour.

The two histological variants of FTC according to the WHO classification are oncocytic and clear-cell types. Oncocytic follicular carcinoma is also called oxyphil or Hürthle-cell carcinoma and is discussed below.

Prognosis

In the case of FTC, the 10-year survival rate varies from 70 to 95 % and for PTC it is a little lower. Prognostic factors that are related to an unfavourable prognosis include age >45 years, oncocytic variant of FTC, neoplasmatic infiltration beyond the thyroid, tumour size >4 cm, and the presence of distant metastases.

Hürthle-Cell Carcinoma

The WHO classification lists Hürthle-cell carcinoma as a variant of FTC, but many authors think that it is a separate pathological entity characterized by a distinct microscopic appearance and clinical behaviour. The oncocytic variant of follicular carcinoma comprises ~5 % of malignant thyroid tumours and, in contrast to FTC, the frequency of nodal metastases in this neoplasm is ~30 %.

Pathogenesis

There is no evidence that the pathogenesis of Hürthle-cell carcinoma is different from conventional FTC, although *H-ras* mutations are found more frequently in this type of tumour than in FTC.

Gross Examination

Macroscopically Hürthle-cell tumours are characteristically brown–mahogany in colour (different from other thyroid tumours) and are encapsulated. The morphological changes within the tumour, such a haemorrhage, cystic areas, infarction, fibrosis and cellular atypia, can be associated, but not exclusively, with a previous FNAB. These changes can also develop independently.

Microscopic Examination

The tumour comprises oncocytic cells, which are the only or the main (at least 75 %) component of the neoplasm. The architecture of this carcinoma can be varied—follicular or solid/trabecular growth patterns. The Hürthle cells have deeply eosinophilic and granular cytoplasm; their nuclei are round and hyperchromatic with prominent nucleoli. Similar to FTC, the differentiation between Hürthle-cell adenoma and carcinoma is based on the same criteria of capsular and/or vascular invasion (*see above*). The malignant tumours are divided into minimally invasive and widely invasive variants.

Prognosis

Patients with Hürthle-cell carcinoma are considered to have a worse prognosis than patients with FTC and PTC. The frequency of lymph node metastases, as well as distant metastases, is higher than in non-Hürthle follicular carcinoma. The lower uptake of radioactive iodine makes treatment of the oncocytic variant of FTC more problematic.

Commentary

R. Kalyani

The chapter on pathology of differentiated thyroid cancers is well structured: the introduction, scope of fine-needle aspiration cytology (FNAC) of thyroid nodules, diagnostic categories, cytological features of papillary carcinoma and follicular neoplasm; the role of frozen section and its limitations are adequately described. However, one should be aware of histological changes after pre-operative FNAC, such as areas along the needle tract of haemorrhage, granulation tissue, cholesterol crystals, adjacent follicular cells showing enlargement and atypia, distortion and disruption of the capsule, all of which give a false picture of capsular invasion during interpretation of follicular neoplasm. Occasionally, squamous cell metaplasia and spindle cell nodules are seen in the needle tract several weeks and months after FNAC. Tumour infarction is common after FNAC, especially in the case of Hürthle-cell neoplasms.

The histopathology of papillary, follicular and Hürthle-cell carcinoma is well presented in terms of their pathogenesis, gross features, microscopic appearance, histological types and prognosis. However, I would like to highlight the following points:

A. *Papillary carcinoma*
  - An increased incidence is also seen in Hashimoto thyroiditis.
  - An occult presentation is common, with the patient presenting with only cervical lymphadenopathy without a clinically detectable lesion/enlargement of the thyroid gland.
  - In the follicular variant of PTC, follicles are irregular, often tubular and branching, with an abortive attempt to form papillae.
  - Psamomma bodies give a clue to the diagnosis.
  - Immunohistochemically, these tumour cells are reactive to thyroglobulin, TTF-1, CK 7+/CK 20, CK 19, high molecular-weight keratin, HBME–1 and RET protein. RT-PCR can be used to detect gene rearrangement in specific RET/PTC.
B. *Follicular carcinoma*
  - This is never occult.
  - Skeletal metastasis is multicentric.
  - Immunohistochemically the tumour cells are reactive to thyroglobulin, TTF–1, low molecular-weight keratin and epithelial membrane antigen, similar to follicular adenoma. However, widespread, strong positivity of galectin-3 supports the diagnosis of follicular carcinoma.
C. *Hürthle-cell carcinoma*
  - CK 14 is emerging as a selective marker for these tumour cells.
  - Tumours with a Ki–67 index of >5 % show aggressive behaviour.

Regarding comments on the Indian situation, in a study performed at our department, entitled *Cancer profile in Department of Pathology of Sri Devaraj Urs Medical College, Kolar: A 10-year study* between January 1997 and December

2006, thyroid cancer constituted ~3.43 % (94 cases) of the total cancers, of which 18 were in males and 76 in females. The majority were papillary carcinomas of the classical type, followed by the follicular variant of PTC, follicular carcinoma and medullary carcinoma. Thyroid cancers are among the top 10 cancers, according to various studies from different parts of India, such as Bangalore, districts of South Karnataka, Hyderabad, Thriruvanthapuram, Dehradun and eastern Rajasthan. This can be attributed to the use of borewell water, which contains a high content of fluorine/iodine, ionizing radiation, and intake of cruciferous and goitrogenic vegetables. It is reported that too much iodine causes papillary carcinoma and iodine deficiency causes follicular carcinoma.

Suggested Reading

Amos KD, Habra MA, Perrier ND. Carcinoma of the thyroid and parathyroid glands. In: Feig BW, Berger DH and Fuhrman GM (eds). *The MD Anderson surgical oncology handbook.* Philadelphia; 2006.
Boerner SL, Asa SL. Biopsy interpretation of the thyroid. In: Biopsy interpretation series. Philadelphia: Wolters Kluwer/Lippincott Williams & Wilkins; 2010
Ito Y, Miyauchi A. Prognostic factors and therapeutic strategies for differentiated carcinomas of the thyroid. *Endocrine Journal* 2009;**56:**177–192.
Koss LG, Melamed MR. *Koss' diagnostic cytology and its histopathologic bases.* Philadelphia: Lippincott Williams & Wilkins; 2006.
Nikiforov YE. Thyroid carcinoma: Molecular pathways and therapeutic targets. *Modern Pathology* 2008;**21:**37–43.
Nikiforov YE, Biddinger PW, Thompson LDR. *Diagnostic pathology and molecular genetics of the thyroid.* Philadelphia: Wolters Kluwer/Lippincott Williams & Wilkins; 2009.
DeLellis RA, Lloyd RV, Heitz PU, Eng C (eds). *Pathology and genetics of tumours of endocrine organs.* (IARC WHO Classification of tumours). IARC Press, Lyon, 2004.
Silverberg SG. Silverberg's Principles and practice of surgical pathology and cytopathology. 4th ed. Churchill Livingstone: Elsevier; 2006.
Syed Z Ali, Cibas ES (eds). *The Bethesda system for reporting thyroid cytopathology. Definitions, criteria and explanatory notes.* Springer Science+Business Media; 2010.

Clinical Evaluation of the Thyroid Gland

3

Artur Komorowski and Andrzej L. Komorowski

In this chapter the authors present the basic rules for clinical evaluation of the thyroid gland.

Introduction

The process of gathering information before establishing a diagnosis and planning the appropriate treatment includes recording the patient's history, performing the physical examination and obtaining the results of laboratory tests. Although medicine now offers a wide range of technically sophisticated instruments that, to an important degree, can help to establish a firm diagnosis, a physician should not forget the first two classical steps: Medical history-taking and physical examination of the patient. Performing these basic steps correctly is especially important because the patient can be saved unnecessary tests and the costs that such tests entail for the healthcare system.

A. Komorowski
Department of Medical Education, Jagiellonian University, Medical College, Krakow, Poland

Department of Radiology, Maria Skłodowska-Curie Memorial Cancer Center and Institute of Oncology, Krakow, Poland

A.L. Komorowski (✉)
Department of General Surgery, Hospital Virgen del Camino, Sanlúcar de Barrameda, Spain
e-mail: z5komoro@cyf-kr.edu.pl

© The Author(s) 2012
F.L. Greene, A.L. Komorowski (eds.), *Clinical Approach to Well-differentiated Thyroid Cancers*, Head and Neck Cancer Clinics,
DOI 10.1007/978-81-322-2568-3_3

Medical History and Physical Examination

Medical History

During medical history-taking, the following key questions should be asked of a patient with thyroid gland complaints:

- Do you have problems with swallowing?
- Do you have breathing difficulties?
- Have you noticed a change in your voice (hoarseness)?
- Have you been coughing lately?
- Have you noticed pain in any area of the neck?
- Have you noticed anything strange or new within your neck?
- Have you noticed a change in your weight?
- Have you noticed that your hands are shaking?
- Have you experienced any unusual sweating?
- Have you or any of your relatives noticed some kind of change in your temper lately? Are you more nervous than usual?
- Have you noticed blood in your sputum?

It is also important to ask the patient for a possible family history of thyroid disorders and previous radiation exposure. Currently, it is estimated that as many as 5 % of all differentiated thyroid cancers can occur in the familial setting. Patients with familial poliposis coli, Cowden disease and Gardner syndrome also have a higher propensity for thyroid malignancies.

It is scarcely worth emphasizing that the information gathered during medical history-taking has to be meticulously noted in the patient's chart.

Clinical features that warrant urgent evaluation and are suspicious of thyroid cancer are also given in Chap. 6 and summarized in Table 6.1.

Physical Examination

Physical examination of the thyroid may be part of an examination of the head and neck, or a stand-alone examination in suspicion of enlargement, inflammation, nodules and other problems.

Before performing a clinical examination of the thyroid the procedure should be described briefly to the patient. The patient should be informed that the neck will be touched from the front and from behind, and that he or she will be asked to drink some water. The patient should be either sitting or standing with a slightly extended neck.

The first step in the clinical examination of the thyroid is inspection. It is best to direct the lighting downward from one side of the patient's chin. The patient should be told to bend the head back slightly so that the neck can be inspected and anatomical landmarks, such as the thyroid cartilage and the cricoid cartilage, can be inspected. The patient should then be asked to take a sip of water, extend the neck slightly and swallow. While he or she does so, movement of the cartilages and the thyroid gland should be noted—these structures should rise with swallowing and then return to their resting positions.

The second step is palpation. It should be remembered that the examiner's hands should be warm during palpation. The neck's landmarks, mentioned above, should be located. The trachea should be inspected for deviation by putting the index finger along one side of the trachea and then along the other side. The space between the sternocleidomastoid muscle and the trachea should be identified; it should be symmetrical on both sides. Thereafter, the isthmus and both lobes of the thyroid should be palpated using only one hand. The second hand can be used to gently retract the sternocleidomastoid muscle. The patient should be asked to swallow so that the isthmus can be felt. If necessary, the patient can be asked to take a sip of water before swallowing.

A posterior approach for palpation of the thyroid is also possible and widely chosen. It is often thought to be the best method. Here, the physician should stand behind the patient and place the hands on the patient's neck so that the index fingers are just below the cricoid cartilage. The patient should be asked to swallow, during which time the isthmus should be palpated. The examination is continued by moving the fingers downwards and laterally.

In both approaches, the size, volume, shape, symmetry and consistency of the thyroid lobes should be noted. Also, any area of tenderness should be looked for and the nodules should be identified and located. It is easier to palpate the thyroid in a long, slim neck than in a short, obese one. Finding the lower borders of the thyroid may be difficult, as it can be partially or totally retrosternal; further extension of the neck may help.

Should the thyroid be enlarged, the final step of the examination is auscultation, using a stethoscope in order to detect a bruit (a murmur due to increased blood flow, similar to a cardiac murmur but of non-cardiac origin) in the lateral lobes.

Common Mistakes

Failure to note in the patient's chart all the pathological information gathered during history-taking and the physical examination.

Commentary

Tahar Benhidjeb

The management of thyroid cancer represents a surgical challenge because of the complex anatomy of the neck region and the gland's close topographical relationship with adjacent organs. Medical history-taking and detailed clinical evaluation are the first and fundamental steps in treatment planning. This chapter describes these cornerstones of thyroid cancer management in a concise way. The approach presented in this chapter corresponds to the way we do medical history-taking and clinical evaluation of patients with thyroid cancer in our institution.

Suggested Reading

Bickley LS, Szilagyi PG (eds). *Bates' guide to physical examination and history taking*. North American Edition. 10th ed. Philadelphia: Lippincott, Williams and Wilkins; 2008
Mazzaferri EL. Management of a solitary thyroid nodule. *N Engl J Med* 1993;**328:** 553–9.
NCCN clinical practice guidelines in oncology. Thyroid carcinoma. V.I.2010.

Imaging in Thyroid Cancer

4

Stephen J. Gwyther

This chapter summarizes current imaging modalities in thyroid cancer.

Introduction

Thyroid cancer is relatively rare. In 2009, it was estimated that 37,200 people (10,000 men and 27,200 women) would be diagnosed with thyroid cancer and that 1630 would die from their disease in 2009 in the United States of America. The incidence is ~10 per 100,000, and >410,000 patients presently suffer from the disease (prevalence).

The vast majority of thyroid cancers are carcinomas—papillary cell carcinomas comprise the majority (75–80 %) followed by follicular cell (10–20 %), medullary (3–5 %) and anaplastic (1–3 %) carcinomas. Other tumour types do occur but are rare and include lymphoma, which may be a primary tumour, often in the setting of pre-existing Hashimoto (chronic lymphocytic) thyroiditis or as part of a generalized lymphoma. Metastases usually arise from primary tumours of the lung, breast and kidney, and squamous cell carcinomas as well as melanomas arise from the head and neck. Sarcomas are rare.

Papillary cell carcinoma has a 95 % 20-year survival rate whereas follicular carcinoma has a 75 % survival rate during the same time span; hence, the low morbidity and mortality rates and the high prevalence compared with many other tumour types. However, medullary cell carcinoma has a less favourable outcome, with a 42–90 % 10-year survival; anaplastic carcinoma has a poor prognosis with <5 % survival at 5 years. Morbidity and mortality rates inevitably rise with the age and stage of the disease.

S.J. Gwyther
Department of Radiology, East Surrey Hospital, Redhill, Surrey, UK
e-mail: GwytherSJ@aol.com

© The Author(s) 2012
F.L. Greene, A.L. Komorowski (eds.), *Clinical Approach to Well-differentiated Thyroid Cancers*, Head and Neck Cancer Clinics,
DOI 10.1007/978-81-322-2568-3_4

27

Factors associated with an increased risk of thyroid cancer include prior irradiation to the neck and a family history of thyroid cancer. Clinical features that suggest malignancy include a firm mass in the neck (particularly in patients aged <20 years and >60 years), a mass that is rapidly enlarging or fixed to adjacent structures, enlarged regional lymph nodes, and vocal cord paralysis.

Against the backdrop of thyroid cancers is the fact that benign thyroid nodules are extremely common and occur in over half of the patients who undergo ultrasound (US) examination of the thyroid gland, whether the examination was performed as a result of a palpable nodule, which occurs in 4–8 % of the population, or discovered by chance at the time of the examination. Only ~7 % of such thyroid nodules are malignant.

High-resolution US of the thyroid gland and neck is unquestionably the investigation of choice for detecting thyroid nodules. However, how can a cancer be distinguished reliably from benign disease in the thyroid?

Imaging of the Thyroid Gland

Ultrasound Examination

High-resolution US examination of the neck undertaken with 7.5–15 MHz probes forms the mainstay of thyroid imaging. However, to confirm a diagnosis of malignancy, cytological or histological proof is required. This is most easily accomplished by performing a US-guided fine-needle aspiration (FNA) of the suspicious nodules. The real question is: can we reliably determine which nodules are likely to be cancerous and therefore merit FNA without subjecting large numbers of patients to unnecessary intervention?

Ultrasound Features Suggesting Malignancy

The ultrasonic features of benign and malignant nodules show considerable overlap. A nodule is a discrete lesion within the thyroid gland that can be distinguished from the normal thyroid parenchyma. The nodule needs to be assessed by means of a grey scale to determine its size; whether it is solid, cystic or mixed; if calcification is present and if it is fine or coarse; if it has a halo or irregular margins; and if colour Doppler US can determine flow patterns within the nodule.

Size

This alone does not predict malignancy; the likelihood of cancer is the same irrespective of size. Other US features including solid hypoechoic lesions containing microcalcifications, poorly defined irregular margins, loss of the halo surrounding the nodule, and increased vascularity within the nodule all suggest malignancy, although the sensitivities and specificities of these findings are extremely variable from one study to another (*see* Table 4.1). However, the European Consensus Group

Table 4.1 US features suggestive of malignancy within thyroid nodules

1. Solid
2. Hypoechoic
3. Microcalcifications
4. Irregular margins
5. Increased vascularity
6. Nodule taller than wider

Fig. 4.1 US scan showing a well-defined nodule in the right lobe of the thyroid gland with multiple microcalcifications (*arrow*). FNA cytology revealed well-differentiated papillary cell carcinoma

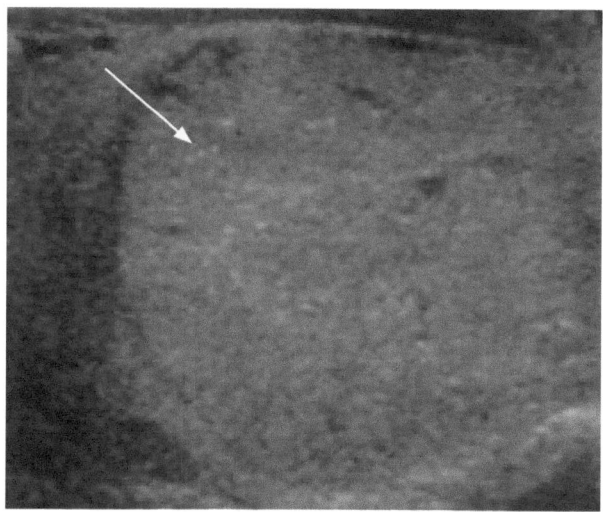

recommends that lesions <1.0 cm be defined as microtumours that need not be biopsied because most cancers are papillary tumours that grow slowly and have an excellent prognosis. Therefore, the risks of surgery outweigh the risks of the tumour, and surgery is not cost-effective. When measuring nodules, the lesion should be measured in its largest diameter, including any halo visible.

Calcification Within a Nodule

Microcalcifications are highly suggestive of malignancy, most commonly in papillary carcinoma, with a frequency of 30–60 %. They appear within nodules as discrete punctuate foci of increased echogenicity without any acoustic shadowing (Fig. 4.1). Coarse macrocalcification within a discrete nodule causes acoustic shadowing and is the most common type of calcification in medullary carcinoma. Benign coarse calcification occurs throughout the gland rather than in specific nodules; peripheral coarse calcification is usually seen in benign multinodular disease, although it may be seen in malignancy.

Composition of the Nodule

Carcinomas and lymphomas both present as solid hypoechoic nodules compared with the surrounding thyroid parenchyma and muscles of the neck, with a sensitivity of 87 % for malignancy. Solid or predominantly solid nodules are more likely to

Fig. 4.2 US scan showing
a cyst with a solid nodule
(*arrow*) within it in the left
lobe of the thyroid gland.
FNA cytology of the solid
nodule demonstrated a
well-differentiated
follicular cell carcinoma

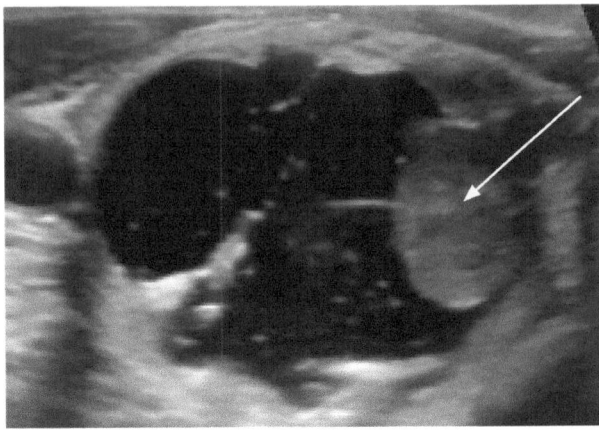

be malignant whereas cystic lesions are extremely unlikely to be malignant. Those
that are partly solid and cystic have some risk for being malignant but not as much
as a solid lesion alone. For this reason, a larger nodule size of 2.0 cm is recommended before FNA is undertaken, although the greater the percentage of the solid
component, the smaller the lesion size before FNA (Fig. 4.2). However, more
recently, the American Association of Clinical Endocrinologists recommended
FNA of all lesions suspicious for malignancy, even if <1.0 cm.

Margins, Contour and Shape

Benign nodules have a well-defined hypoechoic border (halo) but nodules in which
>50 % of the border is not clearly defined may be malignant, although there is consid-
erable overlap between benign and malignant disease. Moreover, a poorly defined,
irregular border suggests direct invasion into the adjacent parenchyma, although this
can be reliably determined only when the tumour is directly seen to invade these structures. Conversely, many benign lesions have poorly defined borders, so this finding
alone is unreliable. The shape of a nodule may predict malignancy. It has been suggested that there is an increased risk of a lesion being malignant when it has a greater
antero-posterior than a transverse diameter, although this remains unproven.

Number of Nodules

Multiple nodules, all of the same echogenicity within a diffusely enlarged gland, need
not undergo FNA as they almost certainly represent a benign multinodular goitre.
However, if the nodules are of differing echogenicity, not all the lesions may be benign.
In one study, almost half of papillary cell carcinomas were found in multinodular
glands. Follicular carcinoma more commonly occurs in a multinodular gland and 20 %
of papillary cell carcinomas are multifocal. If FNA is to be undertaken on a single
nodule, then this should be based on US characteristics, such as calcification, rather
than size of the nodule, although more than one lesion may be biopsied in a multinodular gland. It should be noted that patients at high risk for developing cancer, such as
those who have received previous irradiation to the neck, may be considered for total
thyroidectomy despite a negative FNA because of the high risk of developing cancer.

Vascularity

Colour Doppler studies in malignant nodules demonstrate greater central intrinsic hypervascularity compared with the surrounding thyroid parenchyma. Peripheral flow is more likely to represent a benign lesion, although there is considerable overlap, whereas complete avascularity represents benign disease. However, in the context of a multinodular goitre, colour Doppler studies may demonstrate a specific nodule with central hypervascularity thus targeting this nodule for FNA above others.

Interval Growth of a Nodule

Interval growth is considered a poor indicator of malignancy. It is estimated that >90 % of nodules, both benign and malignant, grow ~15 % in 5 years, although cystic lesions tend not to grow. However, rapidly growing lesions are unusual and FNA or biopsy may be undertaken. Rapidly growing lesions tend to occur in anaplastic carcinomas and lymphomas.

Local Invasion

Direct tumour invasion of the adjacent structures occurs in >36 % of cases and can lead to hoarseness, dyspnoea and dysphagia in rapidly growing aggressive tumours, such as anaplastic carcinoma, lymphoma and sarcoma, which fortunately are uncommon. However, direct tumour invasion also occurs in higher-grade and advanced tumours of any histology.

Lymph Node Metastases

The regional lymph nodes comprise the lateral cervical lymph node chain, which is divided into the internal jugular, posterior triangle and the supraclavicular lymph nodes, and central pre-and paratracheal lymph nodes. Metastatic infiltration occurs in ~19 % of all cases of thyroid cancer. It is most common in papillary carcinoma, occurring in 40 % of adults and 90 % of children with this tumour type. Medullary carcinoma metastasizes early and is found in ~50 % of cases, whereas follicular cancer rarely metastasizes. Lymph node involvement is suggested ultrasonologically by an increase in size. A node measuring >7 mm in its short axis raises the suspicion of malignancy. Other suspicious features include a rounded bulging appearance with replacement of the normal fatty hilum, heterogeneous echo-texture with calcifications, cystic degeneration and irregular margins. Doppler US reveals increased flow throughout the node rather than predominantly at the hilum. In lymphoma, the lesions tend to be markedly hypoechoic and are bulky (Fig. 4.3).

Pitfalls

Lymph nodes can be mistaken for nodules within the thyroid gland if they are cystic or calcified, and this is particularly so when the node appears different from the primary tumour. Cystic metastases are more common in younger patients and one study showed >70 % of patients had predominantly cystic papillary cell carcinoma compared with the primary tumour. Cystic metastases tend to be thick-walled and contain septa and solid nodules.

Fig. 4.3 US scan of the
neck demonstrating two
well-defined hypoechoic
cervical lymph nodes in a
patient with high-grade
primary non-Hodgkin
lymphoma of the thyroid.
A percutaneous core
biopsy of the larger
lymph node was
undertaken and the needle
is demonstrated in the
lymph node (*arrow*)

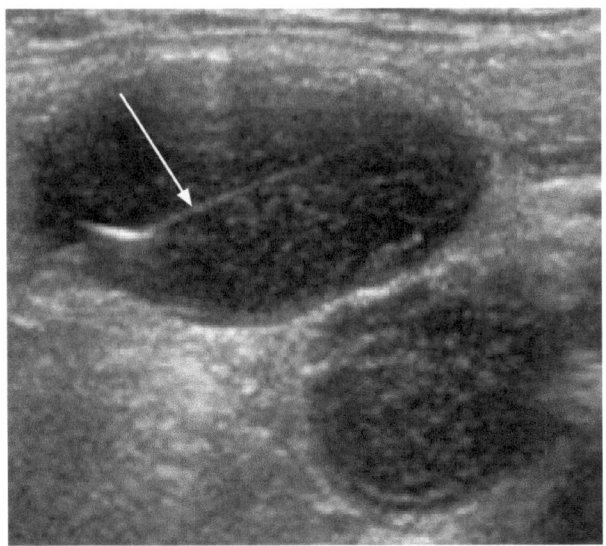

FNA of Thyroid Nodules

A diagnosis of malignancy can only be made categorically with tissue sampled from
the appropriate area. However, benign nodules are very common, while thyroid
malignancy is uncommon, and the mortality and morbidity from small thyroid cancers (<1 cm in size) are low. Utilizing the US criteria given in Table 4.2, US-guided
FNA is preferred to palpation-guided FNA because of a lower false-negative rate
with US-guided FNA (0.6 % versus 3 %). It has a sensitivity of 76–98 %, specificity
of 71–100 %, false-negative rate of 0–5 %, a false-positive rate of 0–5.7 %, and
overall accuracy of 69–97 %. Inadequate specimens may be sampled in 10–20 % of
cases, possibly due to non-standardization of techniques. Side-effects or complications are few. Bleeding may occur, but this is usually minor, even in patients who are
on anticoagulants. The procedure is performed in the outpatient clinic; the patient
lies supine with the head extended. This is achieved by removing the pillow. Local
anaesthetic (1 % lidocaine hydrochloride) can be injected subcutaneously at the
appropriate area, which is necessary if several aspirations are to be undertaken. A
23–27-gauge needle is used and screened into the nodule using real-time US. Once
the tip of the needle is seen in the nodule, the needle can be aspirated using a
5–10 ml syringe. While suction is applied, the needle should be moved back and
forth within the nodule at least five times, the needle tip being viewed continuously
by US. Suction should be stopped before removing the needle from the nodule.
Alternatively, a non-aspiration technique can be undertaken by placing the needle
into the nodule and moving it backwards and forwards several times, allowing some
cellular material to collect in the hub of the syringe by capillary action. The latter is

Table 4.2 Recommendations for thyroid nodules >1 cm in diameter

Nodule type	Recommendation
Solitary nodule with following characteristics:	
Microcalcifications	US FNA >1.0 cm
Solid or coarse macrocalcifications	US FNA >1.5 cm
Mixed solid/cystic	US FNA >2.0 cm
Cystic with mural nodule	US FNA >2.0 cm
Increase in size since previous US	US FNA
Multiple nodules	US FNA of one or more nodules based on
	US criteria

Note: If abnormal lymph node demonstrated, this overrides all other criteria and US FNA of the node is indicated

said to be more useful in hypervascular nodules as it reduces the chance of obtaining a blood-stained specimen, which may render the specimen unsuitable for diagnosis. The narrower the bore of the needle, the greater the chance of obtaining cellular material without it being blood-stained, thus making it suitable for cytological evaluation; a rate of >80 % should be achieved. The specimen obtained should be smeared on glass slides and fixed in 95 % ethyl alcohol. Benign nodules have a higher chance of being inadequate for cytological analysis than malignant nodules. This is said to be more often due to aspiration of cystic, fibrotic or necrotic tissue than to aspiration of the wrong tissue. If the needle tip is visualized, the needle should be in the appropriate nodule.

Cytological Findings
The sample may be non-diagnostic or inadequate, usually because of too few cells being present to make a diagnosis. The commonest causes for this are poor fixation or staining, or excess blood, necrotic material or debris obscuring the cellular material. To be diagnostic, the specimen must contain adequate cellular material and, to make meaningful comparisons, the same criteria as given below need to be applied. Three common criteria are currently in general use.

1. At least five or six groups of well-preserved cells, each containing 10–15 cells
2. Six clusters of benign cells on at least two slides from separate FNA samples
3. Ten clusters of follicular cells, each cluster containing at least 20 cells

Diagnostic samples may be categorized as malignant, indeterminate (suspicious of malignancy) or benign. The first two categories usually require surgical intervention.

Patients with inadequate specimens may have the procedure repeated or may even have a core biopsy, using either an 18- or 20-gauge biopsy needle. Core biopsy provides more histological material, but the complication rate increases significantly, particularly bleeding, in what is already a vascular organ. The author tends to perform core biopsies when there is a high suspicion of lymphoma or on specific nodules after an initial inadequate FNA using a small-bore needle followed by a FNA using a large-bore (19-gauge) needle, which in effect is performing a 'mini' core biopsy.

Computed Tomography Scanning

Computed tomography (CT) scanning plays a limited role in well-differentiated thyroid cancers. A thyroid nodule may be noted incidentally and this may lead to US and US-guided FNA. CT is of greater benefit in aggressive thyroid cancers, particularly poorly differentiated and anaplastic carcinoma and lymphoma, because the tumour has a significantly different and lower attenuation coefficient compared with the normal enhancing thyroid tissue, thereby readily demonstrating local invasion of adjacent structures and tracheal compression (Fig. 4.4). Metastatic disease to the regional lymph nodes and distant metastases, including military lung metastases and lytic bone metastases, are also readily demonstrated. CT- or US-guided biopsy, either FNA or core biopsy, can be undertaken in the context of primary malignancy or in assessing recurrent disease. Occasionally, more than one lesion may require biopsy if the metastatic distribution is unusual or unexpected, or if a second primary tumour is suspected (Fig. 4.5). Core biopsy is undertaken more readily when the tumour is large, of lower attenuation than the normal thyroid tissue and invading

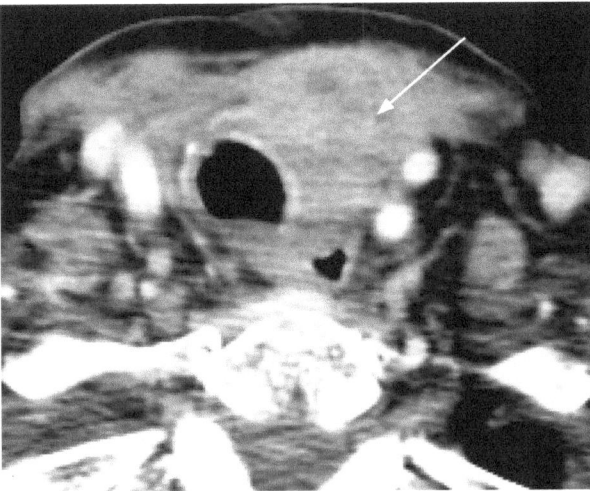

Fig. 4.4 Axial contrast-enhanced CT scan at the level of the thyroid gland showing a large, poorly defined mass arising from the left lobe of the thyroid gland with necrosis, infiltrating the adjacent tissue and structures (*arrow*). This patient had received radiotherapy to the thyroid gland 7 years earlier for a moderately differentiated papillary cell carcinoma of the thyroid gland. Percutaneous core biopsy of this mass demonstrated mixed poorly differentiated papillary cell carcinoma and poorly differentiated squamous cell carcinoma

Fig. 4.5 Axial contrast-enhanced CT scan at the level of the base of the tongue showing a large right-sided para-pharyngeal hypervascular metastasis (*arrow*). Percutaneous core biopsy revealed poorly differentiated metastatic papillary cell carcinoma. Same case as Fig. 4.4

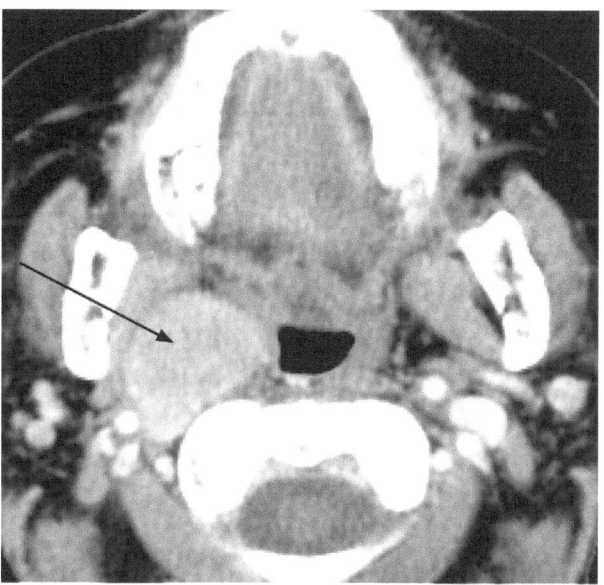

local structures, because it will be less vascular and yield more cellular material. If the histology demonstrates lymphoma, immunohistochemical analysis enables accurate grading and subtyping of the tumour. Where possible, the author uses a 16-gauge biopsy gun to try and obtain optimal tissue for histological analysis. Typically, three separate cores are obtained.

Magnetic Resonance Imaging (MRI)

MRI can demonstrate early invasion of local structures, such as the trachea and the recurrent laryngeal nerve, and abnormal local lymphadenopathy, which may be important in planning surgery in individual cases. However, there is little indication for MRI because CT and US are more cost-effective and capable of achieving similar results.

Whole-Body Isotope Scan Using Iodine 131, and the Use of Serum Thyroglobulin

It is pertinent to mention at this point the role of thyroglobulin and whole-body isotope scan (WBS) using iodine 131 (^{131}I). Thyroglobulin is a protein specific to thyroid tissue where it is synthesized and stored as a precursor to thyroid hormone production. It is also produced by well-differentiated thyroid cancers, particularly papillary cancer. After surgery for a well-differentiated thyroid cancer (and thyroid ablation, should it be undertaken), a baseline thyroglobulin level may be taken.

Thyroid hormone supplements maintain normal thyroid function. A baseline thyroglobulin level >2.0 ng/ml suggests persistent disease and a level below 0.5 ng/ml suggests absence of disease. Subsequent levels that rise with time strongly suggest recurrent disease. The use of thyroglobulin, US scanning and positron emission tomography-CT (PET-CT) has superseded the role of WBS [131]I. A large study of patients who had undergone ablation therapy and were followed with both cervical US and WBS ^{131}I showed a 70 % sensitivity in detecting recurrence with US versus 20 % with WBS. Adding serum thyroglobulin increases the sensitivity in both groups, but more so in the US group.

Positron Emission Tomography-Computed Tomography (PET-CT)

PET-CT plays a role in the detection of recurrent disease in well-differentiated thyroid cancer. Using fluorine 18 F FDG (18-fluoro-deoxyglucose) the sensitivity and specificity for detection of recurrent, well-differentiated thyroid cancer was 68 % and 82 %, respectively; the sensitivity increased with the thyroglobulin level. PET-CT plays a role in the detection of metastatic disease in well-differentiated thyroid cancer in which US of the neck is negative, and has the advantage of imaging the whole body so that distant metastases may be detected. FDG avidity increases with dedifferentiation of recurrent tumour, as glucose metabolism (and glucose transporters [GLUT]) receptor status increases. The main role of PET-CT is to detect local recurrence when the patient has a raised thyroglobulin level but negative neck US or negative ^{131}I WBS. The sensitivity of PET-CT in detecting recurrence varies between 45 % and 100 %, suggesting wide discrepancies in study design, but one large study showed an overall 75 % sensitivity for detecting metastases in well-differentiated thyroid cancer, and an 85 % sensitivity in detecting metastases in those patients with a negative ^{131}I WBS. One major question is, how often does PET-CT alter the clinical management of the patient? Figures between 32 % and 54 % are often quoted but the thyroglobulin and lymph node status have seldom been considered, so the real change in management is likely to be less. The true value of PET-CT remains to be determined, but it may well be of benefit in the small number of patients who develop widespread metastatic disease.

Focal uptake of FDG PET-CT by thyroid lesions may be detected while staging other tumours. One study staging non-small cell lung cancer (NSCLC) detected six cases of focal FDG uptake in the thyroid of 140 patients (4 %). NSCLC is well known to metastatize to the thyroid gland, accounting for >40 % of metastases to the thyroid; FNA revealed four cases of papillary thyroid cancer, one was benign on hemithyroidectomy and one was not biopsied because of the benign appearance on US and CT Focal FDG uptake within the thyroid gland therefore has a high probability of representing a primary thyroid cancer, most likely papillary. The probability increases further when US correlation demonstrates features suggestive of malignancy. However, this needs confirmation because it has a good prognosis whereas metastatic NSCLC has a much worse prognosis.

Conclusion

Thyroid nodules are very common whereas thyroid cancer is relatively rare. US is the imaging modality of choice and although there are no hard and fast rules, certain US features point towards tumours, so these lesions can preferentially undergo US-guided FNA to confirm or refute the diagnosis. Most tumours are papillary and have an extremely good prognosis, but aggressive, anaplastic tumours have a poor prognosis. Thyroid abnormalities may be incidentally detected by other imaging modalities and, depending on the features, if thyroid cancer is suspected, then either US- or CT-guided FNA or biopsy may be undertaken. The trick is to know when to perform a biopsy of the lesion and how far to go, bearing in mind that most well-differentiated papillary cell carcinomas have a 95 % 20-year survival.

Commentary

Josephine N. Rini

The role of ^{131}I whole-body scanning (^{131}I WBS) for surveillance of patients with differentiated thyroid carcinoma (DTC) has declined in the United States of America over the past decade. As discussed by Gwyther, these patients are more often followed with neck ultrasound (US) and serum thyroglobulin (Tg) levels than with ^{131}I WBS. Recombinant human thyroid-stimulating hormone (rhTSH, Thyrogen™), approved by the United States Food and Drug Administration in 1998, as an adjunctive diagnostic tool for serum Tg testing with or without ^{131}I WBS, is one factor that has contributed to this paradigm shift. The subsequent approval of rhTSH, in 2007, for use with ^{131}I ablation has led to a further decrease in radioiodine scanning. In this setting, diagnostic ^{131}I WBS is omitted and a single post-ablation scan is performed. Improved US techniques and standardized criteria for characterizing cervical lymph nodes, as Gwyther notes, as well as efforts to minimize radiation exposure, have also contributed to the decline in radioiodine imaging.

In conjunction with rhTSH stimulation or withdrawal of thyroid hormone, ^{131}I continues to have an important role in patients with treated DTC who have a negative neck US and suspected tumour recurrence based on detectable/rising serum Tg levels. In addition to localizing disease, ^{131}I WBS identifies patients who are likely to benefit from ^{131}I therapy. If ^{131}I WBS is negative, 18-fluoro-2-deoxyglucose (FDG) PET/CT may provide valuable information about the location and extent of disease. The so-called 'flip-flop phenomenon', the finding that DTC is iodine-avid/FDG negative, while dedifferentiated tumours are iodine-negative/FDG avid, provides the basis for this evaluation strategy.

As Gwyther indicates, FDG-PET/CT provides accurate localization of recurrent or metastatic disease in patients with ^{131}I-negative thyroid cancer. It simultaneously provides functional and anatomical information, and has the advantage of surveying the entire body in a single examination. Recently, brain metastases from papillary thyroid carcinoma (PTC) were detected using FDG-PET/CT. Although rare, brain metastases may occur in up to 10–15 % of patients with metastatic PTC who develop new sites of disease. The median survival for patients with brain metastases from thyroid carcinoma (4.7 months) is similar to that reported for patients with brain metastases from other systemic malignancies (4 months). Finally, FDG-PET/CT provides prognostic information because patients with FDG-avid disease have a worse prognosis than those with iodine-avid disease.

Fortunately, most patients with DTC have an excellent prognosis and can be adequately followed with serial neck US and serum Tg levels. For those patients with recurrent or metastatic disease, ^{131}I WBS is useful for determining the extent of disease and for identifying those patients likely to benefit from ^{131}I therapy. For patients with iodine-negative disease, FDG-PET/CT is useful for localizing the disease and providing prognostic information.

Suggested Reading

AACE/AME Task Force on Thyroid Nodules. American Association of Clinical Endocrinologists and Association Medici Endocrinologi medical guidelines for clinical practice for the diagnosis and management of thyroid nodules. *Endocr Pract* 2006;**12**:63–102

Danese D, Sciacchitano S, Farsetti A, *et al*. Diagnostic accuracy of conventional versus sonography-guided fine-needle aspiration biopsy of thyroid nodules. *Thyroid* 1998;**8**:15–21.

Dahnert W. *Radiology review manual*. 5th ed. Philadelphia, Pa: Lippincott Williams & Wilkins; 2003:394–6.

Frates MC, Benson CB, Charboneau JW, *et al*. Management of thyroid nodules detected at US: Society of Radiologists in Ultrasound consensus conference statement. *Radiology* 2005;**237**:794–800.

Grunwald F, Kalicke T, Feine U, *et al*. Fluorine-18 fluorodeoxyglucose positron emission tomography in thyroid cancer: Results of a multicentre study. *Eur J Nucl Med* 1999;**26**:1547–52.

Horner MJ, Ries LAG, Krapcho M, *et al*. (eds). SEER *Cancer Statistics Review*, 1975–2006. National Cancer Institute. Bethesda, MD. http://seer.cancer.gov/csr/1975_2006/, based on November 2008 SEER data submission, posted to the SEER website, 2009

Hay ID, Bergstralh EJ, Goellner JR, *et al*. Predicting outcome in papillary thyroid carcinoma. *Surgery* 1993;**114**:1050–8.

Hoang JK, Lee WK, Lee M, *et al*. US features of thyroid malignancy: Pearls and pitfalls. *RadioGraphics* 2007;**27**:847–60; discussion 861–5.

Imaizumi M, Usa T, Tominaga T, *et al*. Radiation dose–response relationships for thyroid nodules and autoimmune thyroid diseases in Hiroshima and Nagasaki atomic bomb survivors 55–58 years after radiation exposure. *JAMA* 2006;**295**:1011–22.

Jun P, Chow LC, Jeffrey RB. The sonographic features of papillary thyroid carcinomas: Pictorial essay. *Ultrasound Q* 2005;**21**:39–45.

Johnson NA, Tublin ME. Postoperative surveillance of differentiated thyroid cancer: Rationale, techniques and controversies. *Radiology* 2008;**249**:429–44.

Jeong GY, Marom EM, Munden RF, *et al*. Focal uptake of fluorodeoxyglucose by the thyroid in patients undergoing initial disease staging with combined PET/CT for non-small cell lung cancer. *Radiology* 2005;**236**:271–5.

Kessler A, Rappaport Y, Blank A, *et al*. Cystic appearance of cervical lymph nodes is characteristic of metastatic papillary thyroid carcinoma. *J Clin Ultrasound* 2003;**31**:21–5.

Kim MJ, Kim E-K, Park SI, *et al*. US-guided fine-needle aspiration of thyroid nodules: Indications, techniques, results. *RadioGraphics* 2008;**28**:1869–86.

Kwak JY, Kim E-K, Yun M, *et al*. Thyroid incidentalomas identified by 18F-FDG PET: Sonographic correlation. *Am J Roentgenol* 2008;**191**:598–603.

Kim EK, Park CS, Chung WY, *et al.* New sonographic criteria for recommending fine-needle aspiration biopsy of nonpalpable solid nodules of the thyroid. *AJR Am J Roentgenol* 2002;**178:**687–91.

Papini E, Guglielmi R, Bianchini A, *et al.* Risk of malignancy in nonpalpable thyroid nodules: Predictive value of ultrasound and color-Doppler features. *J Clin Endocrinol Metab* 2002;**87:** 1941–6.

Pacini F, Molinaro E, Castagna MG, *et al.* Recombinant human thyrotropin-stimulated serum thyroglobulin combined with neck ultrasonography has the highest sensitivity in monitoring differentiated thyroid carcinoma. *J Clin Endocrinol Metab* 2003;**88:**3668–73.

Shammas A, Degirmenci B, Mountz JM, *et al.* ^{18}F-FDG PET/CT in patients with suspected recurrent or metastatic well-differentiated thyroid cancer. *J Nucl Med* 2007;**48:**221–6.

Staging of Differentiated Thyroid Cancer

5

Wojciech M. Wysocki, Andrzej L. Komorowski,
and Frederick L. Greene

This chapter summarizes the basic information about thyroid cancer staging. Special attention is paid to the AJCC/TNM system.

Introduction

Staging divides patients into prognostic groups to support clinical decisions on the optimal treatment strategy. Appropriate staging also allows comparison of treatment outcomes between medical centres. Differentiated thyroid cancer has many staging systems in use worldwide. It is the authors' opinion that in the absence of a universally accepted staging system, the tumour–node–metastasis (TNM) classification updated regularly by the American Joint Committee on Cancer (AJCC) should be preferred.

TNM Staging System

The current TNM classification (2010) of differentiated thyroid cancer and appropriate stage grouping is presented in Tables 5.1 and 5.2. TNM classification reflects the fact that one of the most important prognostic factors for differentiated thyroid

W.M. Wysocki
Department of Surgical Oncology, Maria Skłodowska-Curie Memorial
Cancer Center and Institute of Oncology, Krakow, Poland

A.L. Komorowski (✉)
Department of General Surgery, Hospital Virgen del Camino, Sanlúcar de Barrameda, Spain
e-mail: z5komoro@cyf-kr.edu.pl

F.L. Greene
Department of General Surgery, Carolinas Medical Center, Charlotte, NC, USA

© The Author(s) 2012   41
F.L. Greene, A.L. Komorowski (eds.), *Clinical Approach to Well-differentiated
Thyroid Cancers*, Head and Neck Cancer Clinics,
DOI 10.1007/978-81-322-2568-3_5

Table 5.1 Definitions of TNM staging for differentiated thyroid cancer

Primary tumour (T)	
Tx	Primary tumour cannot be assessed
T0	No evidence of primary tumour
T1	Tumour ≤ 2 cm in greatest dimension, limited to thyroid
T1a	Tumour ≤ 1 cm, limited to thyroid
T1b	Tumour >1 cm but not >2 cm in greatest dimension, limited to thyroid
T2	Tumour >2 cm but not >4 cm in greatest dimension, limited to thyroid
T3	Tumour >4 cm in greatest dimension limited to thyroid or any tumour with minimal extrathyroid extension (e.g. extension to sternothyroid muscle or perithyroid soft tissues)
T4a	Moderately advanced disease
	Tumour of any size extending beyond thyroid capsule to invade subcutaneous soft tissues, larynx, trachea, oesophagus or recurrent laryngeal nerve
T4b	Very advanced disease
	Tumour invades prevertebral fascia or encases carotid artery or mediastinal vessels
Regional lymph nodes (N)	
Regional lymph nodes include the central compartment, and the lateral cervical and upper mediastinal lymph nodes (see Fig. 7.18)	
Nx	Regional lymph nodes cannot be assessed
N0	No regional lymph node metastasis
N1	Regional lymph node metastasis(-es)
N1a	Metastasis(-es) to Level VI (pretracheal, paratracheal and prelaryngeal/Delphian lymph nodes)
N1b	Metastasis(-es) to unilateral, bilateral, or contralateral cervical (Levels I, II, III, IV or V) or retropharyngeal or superior mediastinal lymph nodes (Level VII)
Distant metastasis(-es) (M)	
M0	No distant metastasis
M1	Distant metastasis(-es)

cancer is age. However, it is important to stress that differentiated thyroid cancers arising in children <10 years of age are more aggressive than thyroid cancers in adults <45 years of age. This fact is not reflected in the current revision of the AJCC/TNM classification.

Other Staging Systems

Other staging systems used for differentiated thyroid cancer include the following classifications: AGES (age, grade, extent, size), AMES (age, metastasis, extent, size), MACIS (metastases, age, completeness of resection, invasion, size) and National Thyroid Cancer Treatment Cooperative Study (size, multifocality, invasion, differentiation, cervical metastases, extracervical metastases). The AGES and AMES classifications divide patients into low-risk and high-risk groups. The mathematical formula to calculate the AGES prognostic score is also in use and is as follows:

Table 5.2 AJCC/TNM stage grouping for differentiated thyroid cancer

Stage	T (Tumour)	N (Node)	M (Metastasis)
Papillary and follicular thyroid cancer (<45 years of age)			
I	Any T	Any N	M0
II	Any T	Any N	M1
Papillary and follicular thyroid cancer (≥45 years of age)			
I	T1	N0	M0
II	T2	N0	M0
III	T3	N0	M0
	T1	N1a	M0
	T2	N1a	M0
	T3	N1a	M0
IVA	T4a	N0	M0
	T4a	N1a	M0
	T1	N1b	M0
	T2	N1b	M0
	T3	N1b	M0
	T4a	N1b	M0
IVB	T4b	Any N	M0
IVC	Any T	Any N	M1

Table 5.3 AGES classification for differentiated thyroid cancer

	Low-risk group	High-risk group
A (age)	Women <50 years of age	Women >50 years of age
	Men <40 years of age	Men >40 years of age
G (grade)	Well differentiated	Poorly differentiated
E (extent)	Limited to thyroid	Infiltration of surrounding tissues and/or distant metastases
S (size)	Diameter <4 cm	Diameter >4 cm

$$\text{AGES prognostic score} = 0.05 \times \text{age} \left(\text{if age} \geq 40 \right) \text{and} + 1 \left(\text{if grade 2} \right),$$
$$+ 3 \left(\text{if grade 3 or 4} \right), + 1 \left(\text{if extrathyroid} \right), + 3 \left(\text{if distant spread} \right),$$
$$+ 0.2 \times \text{tumour size} \left(\text{maximum diameter in cm} \right)$$

Twenty-year survival is 99 % for patients with an AGES prognostic score of ≤3.99, 80 % for an AGES score of 4–4.99, 67 % for an AGES score of 5–5.99, and 13 % for an AGES score of ≥6. Twenty-year survival is 50 % in the high-risk AMES group (Table 5.4) and 98 % in the low-risk AMES group. The clear distinction between low- and high-risk groups allows clinicians to decide which treatment would be suitable for their patient. However, patients' classification according to AMES or AGES criteria has to be also done thoroughly according to the AJCC classification. The AGES (non-mathematical) and AMES staging systems are presented in Tables 5.3 and 5.4, respectively.

Table 5.4 AMES classification for differentiated thyroid cancer

	Low-risk group	High-risk group
A (age)	Women <50 years of age Men <40 years of age	Any age group with distant metastases
M (metastases)	No distant metastases	Distant metastases
E (extent)	Limited to thyroid	Infiltration of thyroid capsule or surrounding tissues
S (size)	Diameter <5 cm	Diameter >5 cm in women >50 years of age or men >40 years of age

Common Mistake

Remember that every case of differentiated thyroid cancer should be staged according to the TNM/AJCC staging system immediately after the diagnosis.

Suggested Reading

Cady B, Rossi R. An expanded view of risk-group definition in differentiated thyroid carcinoma. *Surgery* 1988;**104:**947–53.

Edge SB, Byrd DR, Compton CC, Fritz AG, Greene FL, Trotti A (eds). AJCC cancer staging handbook from the *AJCC cancer staging manual*. 7th ed. New York, Dordrecht, Heidelberg, London: Springer; 2010.

Hay ID, Bergstralh EJ, Goellner JR, *et al.* Predicting outcome in papillary thyroid carcinoma: Development of a reliable prognostic scoring system in a cohort of 1779 patients surgically treated at one institution during 1940 through 1989. *Surgery* 1993;**114:**1050–7.

Sanders LE, Cady B. Differentiated thyroid cancer: Reexamination of risk groups and outcome of treatment. *Arch Surg* 1998;**133:**419–25.

Preoperative Endocrine Management of Differentiated Thyroid Cancer

Barbara Jarząb and Daria Handkiewicz-Junak

This chapter discusses the basic diagnostic procedures that should be performed before a decision is taken to operate on a cancer of the thyroid.

Introduction

Typically, differentiated thyroid cancer (DTC) presents as an asymptomatic thyroid nodule. The patient is referred to an endocrinologist or surgeon to rule out malignancy. The problem in identifying DTC is that <5 % of these thyroid masses are malignant and, furthermore, that the prevalence (3–10 %) in the population of indolent papillary microcarcinomas (≤ 1 cm), which are identified in surgical and autopsy thyroid specimens, is relatively high. Under usual circumstances, these small papillary cancers are not clinically evident, but when serendipitously identified by imaging studies and biopsy, their presence may lead to unnecessary surgery. Thus, identifying a cancer that necessitates a therapeutic intervention in the midst of the many benign nodules is the main challenge in the initial management of DTC. Diagnosis of DTC is followed by establishing a treatment plan, which preferably should be designed by a multidisciplinary team comprising an endocrinologist, surgeon and nuclear medicine physician.

B. Jarząb • D. Handkiewicz-Junak (✉)
Department of Nuclear Medicine and Endocrine Oncology,
Maria Skłodowska-Curie Memorial Cancer Center and Institute of Oncology,
Gliwice Branch, Gliwice, Poland
e-mail: dhandkiewicz@io.gliwice.pl

© The Author(s) 2012
F.L. Greene, A.L. Komorowski (eds.), *Clinical Approach to Well-differentiated Thyroid Cancers*, Head and Neck Cancer Clinics,
DOI 10.1007/978-81-322-2568-3_6

Initial Assessment of a Thyroid Nodule and Diagnosis of Differentiated Thyroid Cancer

Clinical Evaluation

The technique of clinical evaluation of the thyroid gland is described in Chap. 3. Clinical features that warrant urgent evaluation and are suspicious of thyroid cancer are shown in Table 6.1.

Which Thyroid Nodule Should Be Subjected to Fine-Needle Aspiration Biopsy?

Ultrasound of the neck and fine-needle aspiration (FNA) biopsy play a crucial role in the assessment of a thyroid nodule and diagnosis of DTC. Ultrasound helps to distinguish cystic from solid lesions, identify features characteristic of malignant nodules, and detect non-palpable nodules (*see* Chap. 4). Various sonographic characteristics of a thyroid nodule have been associated with a higher likelihood of malignancy (Table 6.2); nevertheless, no single sonographic feature or combination of features is adequately sensitive to identify all malignant nodules. Elastography is an emerging and promising sonographic technique but requires additional validation with

Table 6.1 Clinical features in patients with thyroid nodules warranting urgent differential diagnosis	History of increase in size (rapid growth)
	Family history of thyroid cancer
	History of previous neck irradiation
	Unexplained hoarseness or change in voice
	Cervical lymphadenopathy
	Compression symptoms including dysphagia, dysphonia, hoarseness, dyspnoea and cough
	Stridor
	A nodule that is very firm or hard
	Nodule fixed to adjacent structures
	Very young (<20 of age) or very old (>70 of age) patients

Table 6.2 Ultrasonographic features of a thyroid nodule associated with a higher likelihood of malignancy

Feature	Comments
Hypoechogenicity when compared to normal thyroid parenchyma	Very sensitive but extremely unspecific
Presence of microcalcification	Specificity ~50 %
Irregular infiltrative margins	
Increased intranodular vascularity	As evaluated by Doppler
No 'halo'	

prospective studies. Although these techniques constitute recent developments in imaging, they still suffer from low specificity. Hence, FNA biopsy remains the most accurate and cost-effective method for evaluating a thyroid nodule.

Theoretically, all thyroid nodules should be submitted to FNA biopsy. However, a purely cystic nodule, easily detected during ultrasonography, is highly unlikely to be malignant. Furthermore, a spongiform appearance, defined as aggregation of multiple microcystic components in >50 % of the nodule volume, is highly specific for a benign thyroid nodule. The diagnosis of a 'hot nodule' on scintigraphy of the thyroid (indicated by a serum thyroid-stimulating hormone [TSH] level of <0.1 mU/L) makes the FNA of this nodule unnecessary in most cases (risk of malignancy is <2 %).

Ultrasound frequently discovers nodules that are <1 cm and which usually will not become clinically apparent throughout the patient's life. Thus, FNA biopsy is not routinely recommended for sub-centimetre nodules, unless the patient has a history suspicious of malignancy (e.g. previous radiation exposure, family history of papillary thyroid cancer, or a history of prior thyroid cancer treated with less than total/near-total thyroidectomy), or suspicious ultrasonographic features.

Many patients thought to have a solitary nodule on physical examination are found to have additional nodules on ultrasound examination. This raises the problem of how many nodules should be biopsied in such cases. In a recent study in which 1985 patients underwent FNA of 3483 nodules, it was demonstrated that the likelihood of thyroid cancer in a patient with one or more nodules of >10 mm diameter was independent of the number of nodules. On the other hand, the likelihood of thyroid cancer per nodule decreased as the number of nodules increased. In patients with thyroid cancer and multiple thyroid nodules, the cancer was often unifocal (in 40–48 % of cases) and was diagnosed in the largest nodule in up to 86 % of patients with two nodules but only in 40 % of cases when four or more nodules were present. This observation supports the diagnostic approach in which all thyroid nodules >1 cm should be considered for biopsy. Yet, because cancer in a thyroid gland with multiple nodules is often multifocal, no more than four nodules should be considered for aspiration and the selection should be directed by sonographic risk criteria rather than by nodule size alone. This approach seems reasonable, both in terms of diagnostic costs and side-effects related to FNA biopsy.

Biochemical Examinations for Diagnosis of Differentiated Thyroid Cancer

Measurement of TSH is always performed to exclude thyroid dysfunction but is not useful for differentiating between benign and malignant nodules. Thyroid cancer is seldom the cause of hyperthyroidism, the diagnosis of which indicates a benign hot nodule that can be confirmed with thyroid scintigraphy. Hypothyroidism is infrequent in thyroid cancer and may indicate conditions such as Hashimoto thyroiditis.

Serum thyroglobulin (Tg) is a useful tumour marker, which is used exclusively for the post-surgical follow up of thyroid cancer. Serum Tg levels can be elevated in most thyroid diseases and its preoperative measurement is an insensitive and non-specific test for thyroid cancer.

In contrast, several prospective studies have shown that routine measurement of circulating calcitonin in patients with thyroid nodules may detect C-cell hyperplasia and medullary thyroid cancer at an early stage and hence may contribute to better overall survival. However, most studies rely on pentagastrin stimulation testing to increase the specificity which increases the cost, thereby decreasing the cost-effectiveness of this procedure. The measurement of calcitonin is not recommended in the United States, in spite of a recent analysis suggesting the cost-effectiveness of calcitonin screening; but it is recommended in Europe.

Nuclear Medicine

Thyroid scintigraphy has a limited role in the diagnostic evaluation of thyroid nodules, except in patients with suppressed serum TSH, in whom it should be performed in order to diagnose hyperfunctioning nodules and plan radioiodine treatment.

Currently, positron emission tomography (PET) has no role in the differential diagnosis of DTC. Yet, with the increased use of PET scanning for the staging and surveillance of various malignancies, the phenomenon of the PET-identified thyroid incidentaloma is becoming more prevalent, as evidenced by an increased 18-flourodeoxyglucose (FDG) thyroid uptake in 1–4.8 % of PET examinations. Focal lesions need careful sonographic examination, as 27.8–63 % of these nodules can be malignant.

Additional Diagnostic Procedures

Computed tomography (CT) or magnetic resonance imaging (MRI) should be performed in patients with large tumours to enable a detailed study of the surrounding tissues and mediastinum. Although CT or MRI do not allow differentiation between benign and malignant lesions, infiltration of the surrounding organs or large lymphadenopathy is highly suggestive of malignancy. For more information on imaging studies, *see also* Chap. 4.

Laryngoscopic evaluation is very useful because it allows the diagnosis of vocal cord paresis—another symptom suggestive of thyroid malignancy.

Differential Diagnosis of Differentiated Thyroid Cancer

The main disorders that produce thyroid nodules are shown in Fig. 6.1, but many other factors can cause them, such as tumours metastasizing from other sites. The most common cause of a thyroid nodule is a benign colloid multinodular goitre that often presents as a thyroid nodule diagnosed only on palpation in a gland that does not appear to be enlarged.

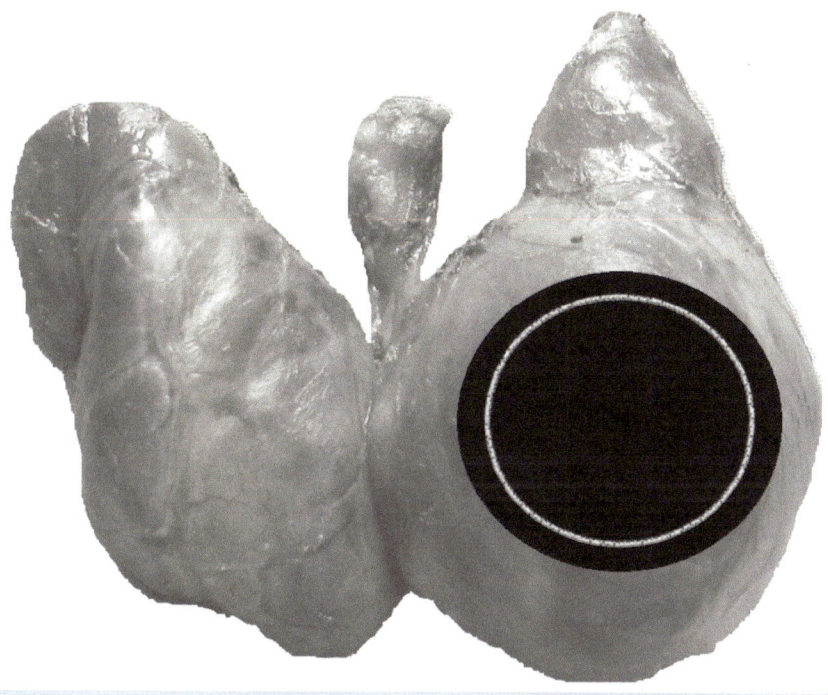

Cancer:	Multinodular goiter:	Cystic lesions:	Other:
– Papillary	– Hyperplastic	– Simple (pure cysts on	– Lymphocytic
– Follicular	nodules	sonography)	thyroiditis
– Poorly	– Colloid nodules	– Haemorrhagic	– Granulomatous
differentiated	– Adenoma	(secondary, on	thyroiditis
– Medullary		sonography often	
– Anaplastic		partially cystic)	
– Metastases from			
different cancers			

Fig. 6.1 The main disorders to be considered in the differential diagnosis of thyroid nodules

Interpretation of Diagnostic Procedures and Initial Approach to Differentiated Thyroid Cancer

On the basis of clinical evaluation and the FNA cytology report, a management plan should be designed, preferably by the multidisciplinary team and in consultation with the patient.

The four main categories that are commonly used to describe FNA cytology: benign, indeterminate (for follicular lesions), malignant and non-diagnostic. Although it is beyond the scope of this chapter to discuss the management of all thyroid nodules, a simplified management decision tree is depicted in Fig. 6.2.

The initial treatment of DTC should be surgery, unless the thyroid is inoperable because of wide infiltration of the surrounding tissues. The extent of the

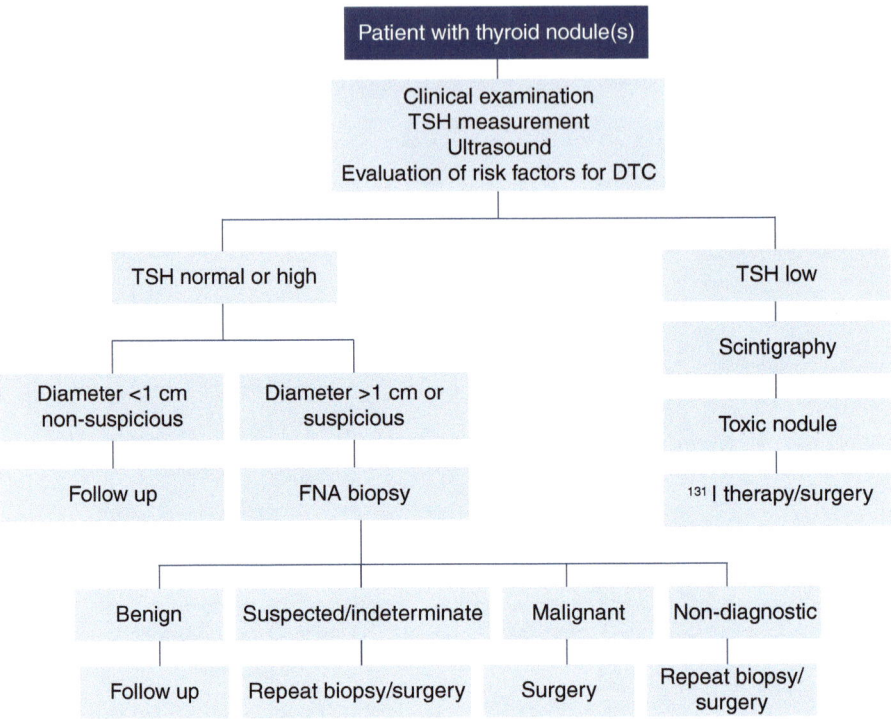

Fig. 6.2 Decision tree in the diagnosis and treatment of thyroid nodules

thyroidectomy, and whether and which lymph node dissection is to be performed, should be discussed by the multidisciplinary team (*see also* Chaps. 7 and 8).

A challenge for both the physician and the patient is to make a management decision after obtaining a diagnosis of indeterminate cytology. This category may sometimes include the 'suspicious for malignancy' group in which malignancy is indicated by some but not all the required features and the smear does not provide sufficient information to make a definitive diagnosis. Surgery, often with intraoperative pathological examination, is the best option in most cases; a second FNA may help to confirm the diagnosis preoperatively. Most doubts are related to those indeterminate cytological findings in which a diagnosis of 'follicular lesion' or 'follicular neoplasm' is made. Cytologically it is impossible to differentiate between follicular adenoma and carcinoma because the diagnosis depends on the absence or presence of capsular or lymphovascular invasion, which can only be determined histologically. A follicular lesion may, in fact, be diagnosed in a follicular variant of papillary cancer (or sometimes, especially if oxyphilic, even in medullary cancer) and also in a hyperplastic nodule or lymphocytic thyroiditis. Thus, the term follicular lesion is preferred over follicular neoplasm by some authors. Approximately 20 % of these indeterminate nodules are malignant but the definitive risk of malignancy depends both on diagnostic criteria and the epidemiological situation. Surgery is recommended to make a definitive diagnosis. However, in elderly patients with chronic, debilitating diseases or in the case of small lesions, careful follow up may be decided upon after a discussion with the patient.

Common Mistake

Among the many benign thyroid nodules, identifying a cancer that necessitates a therapeutic intervention is the main challenge in the initial management of DTC. Currently, ultrasound-guided fine-needle biopsy of the thyroid has a crucial role in differential diagnosis. Other examinations should be performed for rare indications. The most challenging situation arises in those geographical regions where the incidence of nodular goitre is high because of past or present and even mild or moderate iodine deficiency. The highest risk of malignancy is no longer attributed to the diameter of the nodule but to its ultrasound characteristics. Thus, the choice of the biopsied site should be directed by the presence of sonographic risk factors. If multinodular goitre is diagnosed, more than one but probably not more than three or four nodules should be aspirated and a benign result is satisfactory for excluding malignancy. Apart from the presence of some clinical risk factors, such as previous neck irradiation or family history of thyroid cancer, all lesions should be biopsied.

The incidence of small, non-palpable lesions, detectable only by ultrasound, rises up to 50 % with age. Thus, it is unreasonable to take a biopsy of all detected lesions. This should be considered only if at least two sonographic risk criteria are present. Currently, there are no widely accepted molecular criteria that support the differential diagnosis of indeterminate lesions.

The false-positive risk of a definitive cytological diagnosis of thyroid cancer is small (1 %). However, the equivocal character of the cytological diagnosis of follicular lesions has to be accepted, as well as the fact that all required quality criteria cannot always be fulfilled (especially for cystic lesions or in cases of thyroiditis). Nevertheless, a patient with a single thyroid nodule or multinodular goitre should not be referred for thyroid surgery without prior cytological evaluation.

Commentary

Markus Luster

The vast majority of non-palpable and even palpable small nodules are histologically benign and the potential for malignancy is low. Although a growing incidence of DTC has been reported worldwide, the detection of a malignant nodule still resembles 'finding a needle in a haystack' in many cases. The choice of diagnostic procedures is dependent on local circumstances and iodine supply, and the prevalence of goitre. Technetium-based thyroid scanning plays an important role, especially in areas of iodine deficiency, as autonomously functioning nodules rule out malignancy. Sodium-iodine-symporter expression in DTC is supposed to be

1000-fold lower than in benign thyroid tissue. At least in the hands of our team, only hypofunctioning nodules merit FNA on account of the high rate of false-positive results ('follicular neoplasia') in 'hot nodules'. Borget et al. showed that the cost of FNA depends on cytopathologist performance and unsatisfactory specimen rate. The authors foresee that in the future, routine ultrasound guidance and on-site assessment of cytopathological adequacy would help reduce costs.

The ultimate initial test for thyroid examinations remains neck ultrasound because of its easy accessibility and effectiveness; the main drawback is investigator dependency. The use of high-resolution ultrasonography is generally considered the first choice for the evaluation of thyroid size and morphology. It is much more reliable than palpation of the gland (which has an accuracy of only ~40 %) and reduces the interobserver variation. Sonographic features as predictors of malignancy have been widely reported and debated; the presence of multiple criteria increases specificity at the cost of sensitivity.

The number of incidental findings, i.e. 'hot spots' in the thyroid region, has increased with the advent of PET/CT. A systematic use of FDG-PET scanning for screening reasons cannot be recommended because of the lack of specificity, especially in areas with a high prevalence of goitre.

Suggested Reading

Belfiore A, La Rosa GL, Padova G, *et al.* The frequency of cold thyroid nodules and thyroid malignancies in patients from an iodine-deficient area. *Cancer* 1987;**60:**3096–102.

Bonavita JA, Mayo J, Babb J, *et al.* Pattern recognition of benign nodules at ultrasound of the thyroid: Which nodules can be left alone? *AJR Am J Roentgenol* 2009;**193:**207–13.

Cheung K, Roman SA, Wang TS, *et al.* Calcitonin measurement in the evaluation of thyroid nodules in the United States: A cost-effectiveness and decision analysis. *J Clin Endocrinol Metab* 2008;**93:**2173–80.

Costante G, Meringolo D, Durante C, *et al.* Predictive value of serum calcitonin levels for preoperative diagnosis of medullary thyroid carcinoma in a cohort of 5817 consecutive patients with thyroid nodules. *J Clin Endocrinol Metab* 2007;**92:**450–5.

Cooper DS, Doherty GM, Haugen BR, *et al.* Revised American Thyroid Association management guidelines for patients with thyroid nodules and differentiated thyroid cancer. *Thyroid* 2009;**19:**1167–214.

Eloy JA, Brett EM, Fatterpekar GM, *et al.* The significance and management of incidental [18 F] fluorodeoxyglucose-positron-emission tomography uptake in the thyroid gland in patients with cancer. *AJNR Am J Neuroradiol* 2009;**30:**1431–4.

Frates MC, Benson CB, Doubilet PM, *et al.* Prevalence and distribution of carcinoma in patients with solitary and multiple thyroid nodules on sonography. *J Clin Endocrinol Metab* 2006;**91:**3411–17.

Pacini F, Pinchera A, Giani C, *et al.* Serum thyroglobulin in thyroid carcinoma and other thyroid disorders. *J Endocrinol Invest* 1980;**3:**283–92.

Pacini F, Schlumberger M, Dralle H, *et al.* European consensus for the management of patients with differentiated thyroid carcinoma of the follicular epithelium. *Eur J Endocrinol* 2006;**154:** 787–803.

Rago T, Santini F, Scutari M, *et al.* Elastography: New developments in ultrasound for predicting malignancy in thyroid nodules. *J Clin Endocrinol Metab* 2007;**92:**2917–22.

Ron E, Lubin JH, Shore RE, *et al.* Thyroid cancer after exposure to external radiation: A pooled analysis of seven studies. *Radiat Res* 1995;**141**:259–77.

Shie P, Cardarelli R, Sprawls K, *et al.* Systematic review: Prevalence of malignant incidental thyroid nodules identified on fluorine-18 fluorodeoxyglucose positron emission tomography. *Nucl Med Commun* 2009;**30**:742–8.

Sippel RS, Caron NR, Clark OH. An evidence-based approach to familial nonmedullary thyroid cancer: Screening, clinical management, and follow-up. *World J Surg* 2007;**31**:924–33.

Surgical Treatment of Thyroid Cancer

Marcin Barczyński

Introduction

The purpose of this section is to provide a brief summary of the optimal surgical management for well-differentiated thyroid cancer, as well as to present a step-by-step technique of safe total thyroidectomy with central lymph node dissection. It is also aimed to outline a clinical application of recent advances in thyroid surgery: Intraoperative recurrent laryngeal nerve (RLN) monitoring and intraoperative parathyroid hormone (iPTH) assay.

Extent of Surgery

The primary treatment of well-differentiated thyroid cancer is surgical ablation. Fine-needle aspiration cytology (FNAC), as a diagnostic tool of thyroid cancer, enables treatment to be planned and discussed with the patient prior to surgery. The extent of surgery for patients with high-risk papillary thyroid carcinoma (PTC) is scarcely debatable, with most clinicians agreeing on total (the removal of both thyroid lobes, isthmus and pyramidal lobe) or near-total thyroidectomy (a complete removal of thyroid lobes leaving behind only the smallest amount of thyroid tissue [significantly <1 g] to protect the RLNs). However, the ideal extent of surgery for low-risk, small, intrathyroidal, well-differentiated PTCs remains controversial. It is generally agreed that in the surgical management of well-differentiated thyroid cancer the rule should be applied of increasing the extent of surgery along with an increasing risk of thyroid cancer, as well as an increasing stage of the disease. Most

M. Barczyński
Department of Endocrine Surgery, 3rd Chair of General Surgery,
Jagiellonian University, Medical College, Krakow, Poland
e-mail: marbar@mp.pl

© The Author(s) 2012
F.L. Greene, A.L. Komorowski (eds.), *Clinical Approach to Well-differentiated Thyroid Cancers*, Head and Neck Cancer Clinics,
DOI 10.1007/978-81-322-2568-3_7

surgeons and endocrinologists recommend thyroid lobectomy for patients with occult PTCs (<1 cm) and for patients with minimally invasive follicular thyroid cancers (FTCs), because these patients have little risk of dying from these tumours. Lobectomy with isthmectomy is also the treatment of choice for non-compliant patients who will not take thyroid hormone and for those who do not have access to thyroid hormone. Other surgeons recommend a similar approach for patients determined to be at low risk by the AGES (age, grade, extent, size) or AMES (age, metastases, extent, size) classification (*see* Chap. 5), and more extensive resection (near-total or total) for high-risk patients and for patients with bilateral tumours. It is important to stress that subtotal thyroidectomy, leaving >1 g of tissue with the posterior capsule on the uninvolved side, is an inappropriate operation for thyroid cancer. However, opponents of total thyroidectomy have argued that the overall survival rates for PTC are excellent regardless of the extent of surgery, that local recurrences can usually be cured with surgery, that multifocality has questionable clinical significance, and that total thyroidectomy exposes the patient to the risks of permanent hypoparathyroidism and bilateral RLN injury. On the other hand, it is well known that multiple aspects of postoperative treatment and follow up are facilitated by more extensive thyroidectomy, even in low-risk patients. The rationale for total thyroidectomy includes several issues, including the following:

- PTC has been found to be multicentric in 30–80 % of cases and bilateral in ~60 % of patients. Thus, adequate surgical clearance of disease is available only with total thyroidectomy.
- Bilateral thyroid resection obviates the need for completion thyroidectomy, which is usually associated with a higher risk of complications.
- When thyroid tissue is removed, postoperative ^{131}I scanning and ablative therapy of microscopic disease is more effective.
- Serum thyroglobulin (Tg) levels are rendered more sensitive for detecting recurrent or persistent disease after total thyroidectomy.
- In addition, a small risk of well-differentiated thyroid cancer becoming an undifferentiated thyroid cancer is decreased by total thyroidectomy.
- More extensive thyroidectomy is associated with a lower recurrence rate and improved survival.
- Moreover, the RLN palsy rate and prevalence of permanent hypoparathyroidism is not increased after total thyroidectomy (if performed by an experienced thyroid surgeon in a high-volume centre) when compared with more limited thyroid resection.

Recent data from the National Cancer Data Base (NCDB) demonstrate that the use of total thyroidectomy for PTC has increased over the past 20 years, from 70.8 % in 1985 to 90.8 % in 1992, reaching a plateau at ~90 % since 1993. Bilimoria et al. examined >90,000 patients with PTC of ≥1 cm from the NCDB from 1985 to 2003. Patients treated at low-volume and community hospitals were less likely to undergo a total thyroidectomy than patients treated at high-volume or National Comprehensive Cancer Network (NCCN)/National Cancer Institute (NCI) centres. Thus, differences

Table 7.1 Indications for total thyroidectomy

Indeterminate FNAC, i.e. follicular neoplasm or Hürthle cell neoplasm
Tumours >4 cm
Marked atypia seen on biopsy
Biopsy reading 'suspicious for papillary carcinoma'
Family history of thyroid carcinoma
History of radiation exposure
Bilateral nodular disease
Patient's wish

FNAC fine-needle aspiration cytology

in the use of total thyroidectomy can be related to patient, tumour and hospital factors, and possibly reflect disparities in access to care.

Much of the debate with respect to the extent of surgery for thyroid cancer has been addressed recently in the Revised American Thyroid Association Management Guidelines for Patients with Thyroid Nodules and Differentiated Thyroid Cancer. These guidelines, in fact, support the concept that total or near-total thyroidectomy should be utilized in most patients with well-differentiated thyroid cancers. Because of the risk of malignancy approaching 20 %, total thyroidectomy should be indicated in patients who meet the criteria given in Table 7.1.

Those patients should also undergo total or near-total thyroidectomy who have bilateral nodular disease with indeterminate nodules, or those who prefer to undergo bilateral thyroidectomy to avoid the possibility of requiring future surgery on the contralateral lobe. However, for patients with an isolated, indeterminate solitary nodule who prefer a more limited surgical procedure, thyroid lobectomy can be recommended as an initial surgical approach.

Total or near-total thyroidectomy should be recommended if the following criteria are met:

1. The primary thyroid carcinoma is >1 cm.
2. Contralateral thyroid nodules are present.
3. Regional or distant metastases are present.
4. The patient has a personal history of radiation therapy to the head and neck.
5. The patient has a first-degree family history of well-differentiated thyroid cancer.

Older age (>45 years) may also be a criterion for recommending near-total or total thyroidectomy even with tumours of <1.5 cm because of higher recurrence rates in this age group. An increased extent of primary surgery may improve survival not only for high-risk patients but also for low-risk patients. Bilimoria et al. showed in a study of over 50,000 patients with PTC that total thyroidectomy significantly improved recurrence and survival rates in those with tumours of >1.0 cm. When examined separately, even patients with 1.0–2.0 cm tumours who underwent lobectomy had a 24 % higher risk of recurrence and a 49 % higher risk of mortality from thyroid cancer ($p = 0.04$ and $p < 0.04$, respectively). Other studies have also shown that the rates of recurrence are reduced by total or near-total thyroidectomy among low-risk patients.

Central Compartment Lymph Node Clearance

Regional lymph node metastases are present at the time of diagnosis in 20–90 % of patients with PTC and in a much lesser proportion of patients with FTC. The recently published SEER (Surveillance, Epidemiology, and End Results) registry study concluded that cervical lymph node metastases conferred an independent risk of decreased survival, but only in patients with follicular cancer and those with papillary cancer aged >45 years. Also, the risk of regional recurrence is higher in patients with lymph node metastases, especially in those patients with multiple metastases and/or extracapsular nodal extension.

In many patients, lymph node metastases in the central compartment do not appear abnormal preoperatively with imaging or by inspection at the time of surgery. Although some lymph node metastases may be treated with ^{131}I, several treatments may be necessary, depending upon the histology, size and number of metastases. Central compartment dissection (therapeutic or prophylactic) can be achieved with low morbidity in experienced hands. Thus, comprehensive bilateral central compartment node dissection may improve survival and reduce the risk for nodal recurrence. However, a few studies of central compartment dissection have demonstrated higher morbidity primarily RLN injury and transient hypoparathyroidism, with no reduction in the rates of undetectable or low Tg levels and recurrence.

It is generally agreed that therapeutic central compartment (level VI) neck dissection for patients with clinically involved central or lateral neck lymph nodes should accompany total thyroidectomy. Prophylactic central compartment neck dissection (ipsilateral or bilateral) may be performed in patients with PTC with clinically uninvolved central neck lymph nodes, especially for advanced primary tumours (T3, T4). On the other hand, near-total or total thyroidectomy without prophylactic central neck dissection may be appropriate for small (T1, T2), non-invasive, clinically node-negative PTCs and most follicular cancers. Particularly in the case of patients with small, non-invasive, apparently node-negative tumours, the risk/benefit ratio may favour simple near-total thyroidectomy with close intraoperative inspection of the central compartment, with compartmental dissection being performed only in the presence of obviously involved lymph nodes. This approach may increase the chance of locoregional recurrence, but may be safer for less experienced thyroid surgeons.

Sentinel Lymph Node

The use of sentinel lymph node biopsy has been popularized for the treatment of melanoma and breast cancer since the early 1990s. The technique finds its place where formal lymph node dissection is associated with significant morbidity, such as in the groin or axilla. Sentinel lymph node biopsy has recently been utilized to map tumour lymphatics in patients with well-differentiated thyroid cancer. Currently, controversy centres around the feasibility and future role of this technique in the management of patients with well-differentiated thyroid cancer. Sentinel lymph node biopsy can be used in thyroid cancer patients utilizing a vital dye technique, a radiotracer technique, and a combination of both. In the current literature, the average rate of sentinel node identification is 91 % (range 66–100 %) and, when identified, the sentinel node accurately predicts the disease status of the neck in most patients (range 80–100 %). Limitations to carrying out a sentinel node biopsy in thyroid cancer patients include staining of the parathyroid glands, identification of lymph nodes draining into the mediastinum, and the 'shine through' effect, i.e. high activity of the background, especially problematic in the central neck compartment where the lymph nodes are located in close proximity to the thyroid. In addition, skip metastases (lateral compartment involvement without central compartment metastasis) can be a problem, particularly in patients with thyroid cancer situated within the superior poles of the thyroid lobes, or in cases of bilateral and/or multicentric tumours. Some data suggest that sentinel node biopsy is an accurate and non-invasive means of identifying subclinical lymph node metastasis. This technique can be used as an intraoperative guide when determining the extent of surgery necessary in cervical level VI by virtue of the fact that negative sentinel lymph nodes correlate strongly with a negative central compartment involvement. The benefit of sentinel lymph node biopsy has been recently questioned, as non-invasive imaging with high-resolution ultrasound can produce similar results. Thus, sentinel lymph node biopsy is technically feasible but its clinical utility in the management of patients with well-differentiated thyroid cancer seems to be limited.

Completion Thyroidectomy

Completion thyroidectomy may be necessary when the diagnosis of malignancy is made after lobectomy for an indeterminate or non-diagnostic biopsy. The most common indication for completion thyroidectomy is a frozen section analysis of a thyroid lesion that is interpreted as benign follicular adenoma (this is one of the reasons why frozen section is not encouraged; see Chap. 2 for details). On a subsequent final pathology report, areas of invasion are identified and the diagnosis is changed to follicular carcinoma. Some patients with malignancy may require completion thyroidectomy to provide complete resection of multicentric disease, and to allow ^{131}I therapy. This includes all patients with thyroid cancer except those with small (<1 cm), unifocal, intrathyroidal, node-negative, low-risk tumours. Therapeutic central neck lymph node dissection should be included if the lymph nodes are clinically involved. Due to a dearth of prospective studies, data are lacking to demonstrate that the completion thyroidectomy has any impact on recurrence or survival. Thus, the decision of whether to operate should be individualized. If the patient is in the low-risk group (e.g. a 35-year-old woman with a 1 cm minimally invasive follicular cancer) it is reasonable to maintain the patient on thyroxine suppression and not perform completion thyroidectomy. On the other hand, if the patient is in the high-risk group, completion thyroidectomy should be undertaken.

The surgical risks of two-stage thyroidectomy (lobectomy followed by completion thyroidectomy) are similar to those of a near-total or total thyroidectomy. However, the risk of completion thyroidectomy after subtotal thyroidectomy is much higher and, if required, this should be attempted no later than 2–3 days after the initial operation to avoid difficulties in dissection within the inflamed tissues, or at least 8–12 weeks later when recognition of vital anatomical details is easier.

Technique of Thyroidectomy

The safety of thyroidectomy is a major concern for both patients and physicians. A good thyroid operation presents a greater challenge and requires more technical precision and skill than an adrenalectomy or removal of any gastrointestinal endocrine tumour. The accepted rate of permanent hypoparathyroidism and permanent vocal palsy is between 1 and 2 % for primary thyroid operations. Surgeons performing thyroid surgery must learn how to perform a safe total thyroidectomy by training with an experienced thyroid surgeon. There is strong evidence that the complication rates are higher after total thyroidectomy when the surgery is performed by surgeons who have not specialized in thyroid surgery. Population-based volume-outcome studies have suggested that the risk of nerve injury and hypocalcaemia is significantly higher in low-volume centres. Unfortunately, at least 50 % of all thyroid operations are performed in the USA and in Europe by low-volume thyroid surgeons (<50 thyroid operations per year). Total thyroidectomy is an operation that always involves a controversy related to morbidity due to RLN and parathyroid injury. A 'casual' thyroid surgeon can be exposed to the distinct possibility of medical malpractice litigation in case of any permanent morbidity after total thyroidectomy for a low-risk thyroid cancer. However, more recent data showed that surgeons who have completed a well-designed training programme and who have become proficient in total thyroidectomy as trainees will remain proficient despite practising in low-volume centres. Achieving a low morbidity rate demands meticulous attention to operative technique and anatomical detail. This observation underlines that operative skills and experience determine the complication rates to a greater extent than the type of thyroid resection (e.g. total thyroidectomy versus near-total thyroidectomy) (Table 7.2).

Table 7.2 General principles applicable to all thyroid operations

Good exposure of the thyroid gland
Proper identification of vital anatomical structures (parathyroid glands, laryngeal nerves)
Surgery in a dry operative field without bleeding (suction should be avoided)
Wise use of energy-based tools for haemostasis and tissue dissection (e.g. diathermy, ultracision)

Fig. 7.1 Patient's position on the table

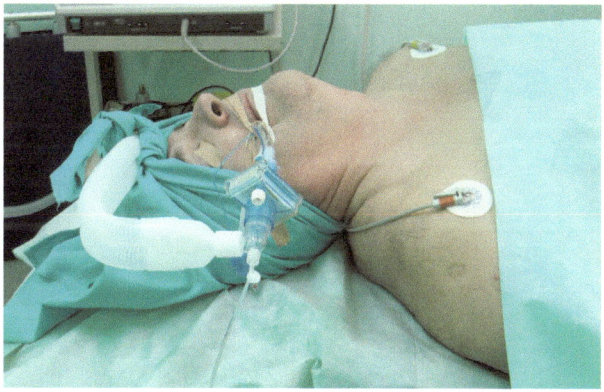

Patient Positioning for Surgery

Virtually all patients with thyroid cancer undergo surgery under general anaesthesia with endotracheal intubation. This gives more comfort to the surgeon and protects the airway and lungs of the patient from aspiration. Prior to any thyroid operation, the patient must be positioned appropriately, with the neck hyperextended (Fig. 7.1). This manoeuvre allows the protrusion of the inferior thyroid lobes if they are localized in a substernal position. A pad or a set of folded sheets should be placed parallel to the spinal column. This pad should be wide enough to prevent the patient from rolling off but narrow enough to allow the shoulders to fall posteriorly. A doughnut pad should be placed behind the patient's head to keep it from moving. The degree of hyperextension is often limited in older patients. Pharmacological muscle relaxation is helpful to achieve optimal positioning. Slight elevation of the head of the operating table, up to 10°, helps in decreasing venous engorgement. Surgical drapes should be attached to the skin so that they conform to the patient's neck and leave uncovered the entire anterior aspect of the neck from the chin to the suprasternal notch and from the posterior aspect of one sternocleidomastoid muscle to the other.

Planning an Incision

A transverse skin incision is made ~2–3 cm above the sternal notch. The incision provides a direct approach to the thyroid gland and its adjacent structures while allowing optimal postoperative cosmetic results (Fig. 7.2). Placing an incision too low in the neck, just above the clavicular heads, should be avoided, particularly as these incisions tend to spread. A higher location of the incision in the neck produces a more satisfactory appearance. If possible, the incision incorporates wrinkle lines for optimal cosmetic healing. Incisions have a tendency to fall caudally with advancing age of the patient. Many surgeons outline the incision by placing a suture across a crease line in the neck, creating pressure, and then making the incision in the depressed line. Others prefer to carefully mark the midline and draw a slightly

Fig. 7.2 Planning an
incision

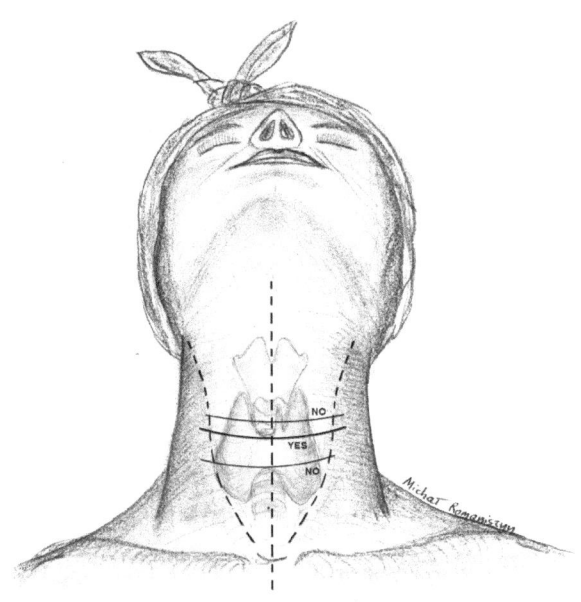

upward curved line across the neck at a level that is measured and marked by a pen. The length of the skin incision depends generally on the size of the goitre, and can approach the medial borders of the sternocleidomastoid muscles, but it can be lengthened in parallel to the sternocleidomastoid muscle border if lateral neck dissection is planned. Small incisions should be made in patients with small thyroid nodules or goitres, and in patients who have a thin, flexible neck.

Thyroid Exposure and Dissection

The skin incision is carried through the subcutaneous fat and platysma muscle. Superior and inferior flaps are dissected in an avascular plane beneath the platysmal layer (Figs. 7.3, 7.4, and 7.5). The anterior jugular veins are identified and divided if crossing the midline. Good exposure is obtained by separating the strap muscles (sternohyoid and sternothyroid) in the avascular midline raphe from the thyroid cartilage to the sternal notch. Just beneath this plane the isthmus of the thyroid can be identified in the midline lying on the anterior aspect of the trachea and each of the lobes laterally. Blunt finger dissection can be used to separate the sternohyoid muscles from the thyroid capsule. However, because the sternothyroid muscles are in a deeper and more lateral position than the sternohyoid muscles, they must be separated off the thyroid capsule to allow lateral exposure of the thyroid.

If the thyroid tumour is large, a complete transverse division of the strap muscles should be made in their upper third to minimize denervation (Fig. 7.6). The sternohyoid muscles are repaired at the end of the operation. It is common for malignant

Fig. 7.3 Mobilization of the upper flap (skin, subcutaneous fat and platysma muscle are mobilized as one layer)

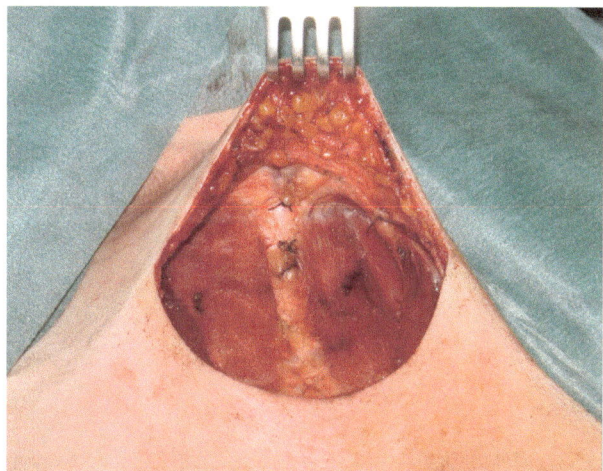

Fig. 7.4 Mobilization of the lower flap to the level of the clavicles and suprasternal notch

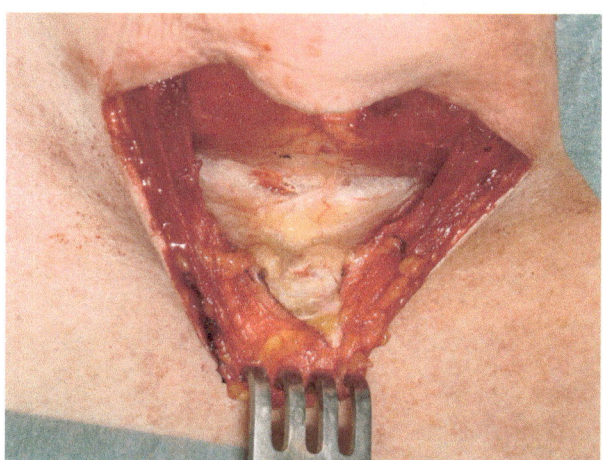

disease to infiltrate the muscles. In such a case, muscles adherent to the tumour should be resected *en bloc* with the thyroid gland.

The sternothyroid muscle should be dissected free from the thyroid gland by pushing gently posteriorly and medially on the thyroid, and pulling laterally and anteriorly on the muscles.

The thyroid gland is exposed once the strap muscles are dissected in the midline or divided transversely (Fig. 7.7). Dissection of the pyramidal lobe can be conveniently done either at this stage of the operation or later (Fig. 7.8). Mobilization of the thyroid lobe towards the midline facilitates identification of the middle thyroid vein and inferior thyroid artery (Fig. 7.9). Once identified, the middle thyroid vein is divided and ligated. This vessel drains directly into the jugular vein. Failure to ligate it securely may cause haemorrhage, which can make it difficult to identify

Fig. 7.5 Both upper and lower flaps are mobilized and strap muscles are exposed

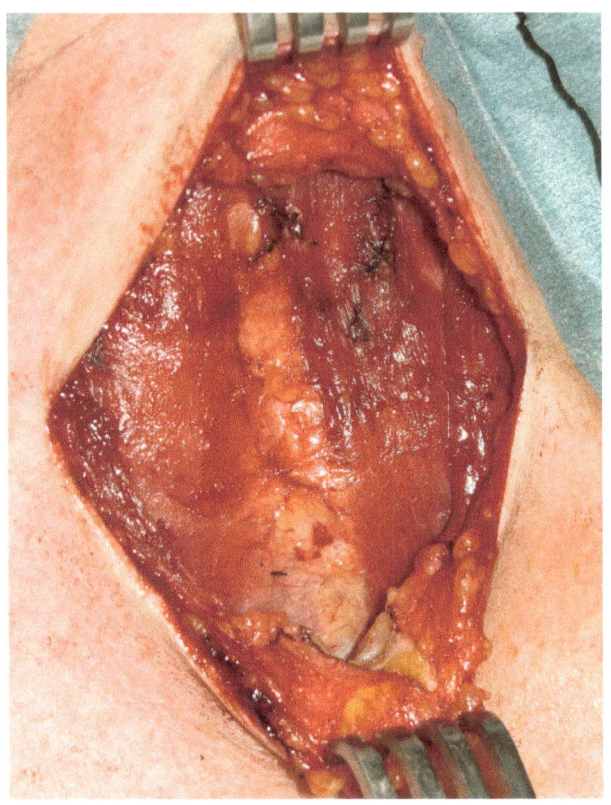

Fig. 7.6 Transverse division of the left strap muscles at the upper third

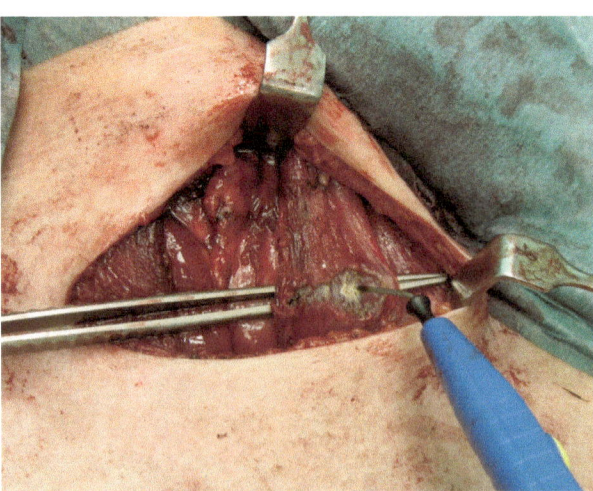

Fig. 7.7 Once the strap
muscles are dissected in
the midline or divided
transversely the thyroid
gland is exposed

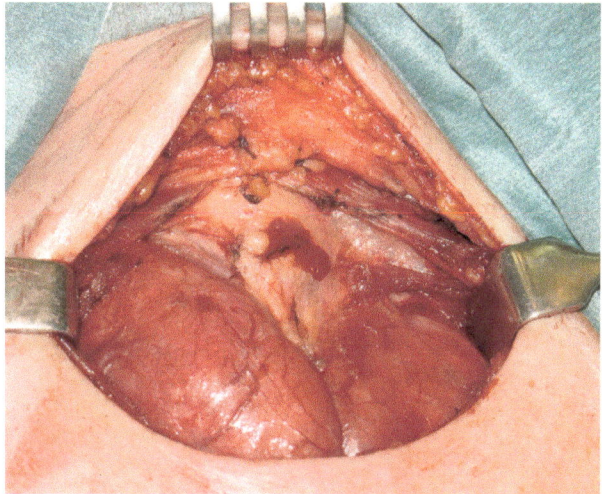

Fig. 7.8 Dissection of
the pyramidal lobe

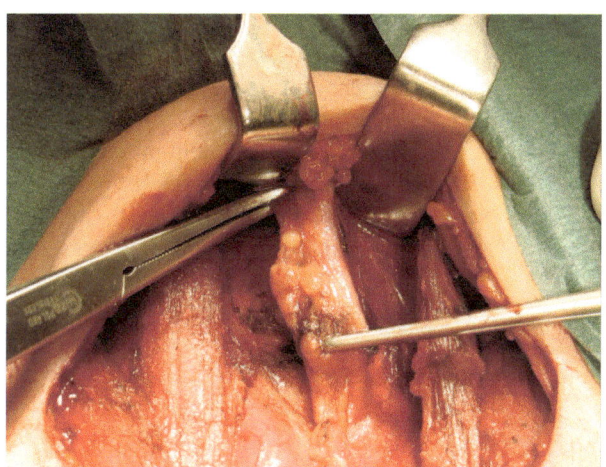

other vital anatomical structures within the neck. The tissues adjacent to the thyroid
are then gently pushed away or dissected from the thyroid gland to expose the inferior thyroid artery.

The next step is to divide the vessels of the superior pole of the thyroid lobe. When
retraction of the thyroid lobe is done in a caudal and lateral direction, tension can be
placed on the superior pole vessels so that they can be identified. The RLN enters the
most caudal portion of the cricothyroid muscle at a position below the upper portion
of the thyroid lobe and below the inferior lobe of the thyroid cartilage. Thus, mobilization in this area can be done quickly and safely. It is helpful to divide the cricothyroid
branch of the superior thyroid artery to gain access to the space between the cricothyroid muscle and superior pole vessels. Medial to the upper pole vessels is the external

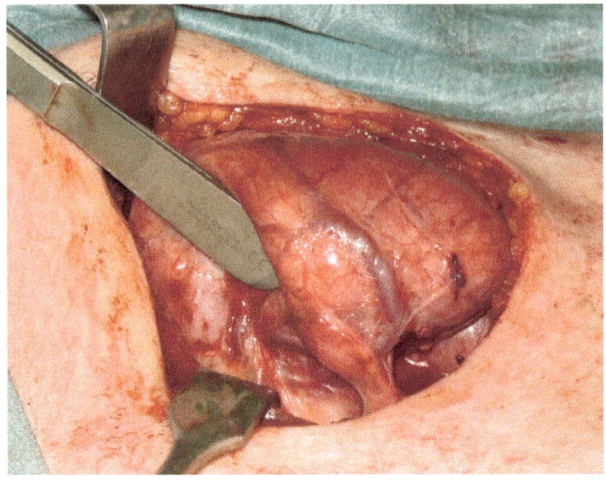

Fig. 7.9 Mobilization of the right thyroid lobe towards the midline facilitates identification of the right inferior thyroid artery (the middle thyroid vein was divided first)

branch of the superior laryngeal nerve, which runs along the cricothyroid muscle in most patients (Fig. 7.10). To avoid injury to this nerve, which controls the tension of the vocal cords, the superior pole vessels should be divided individually as close as possible to the point where they enter the thyroid gland (Fig. 7.11). The nerve can sometimes be seen, but is not visible in most instances. The author prefers to divide the superior pole vessels initially because this manoeuvre increases the mobility of the thyroid lobe, allowing for an easier approach to the superior parathyroid gland and the RLN, which are usually localized deeper in the neck within the tracheo-oesophageal (TE) groove and behind the Berry ligament. At this stage of the operation, as the thyroid is retracted medially, gentle dissection is used to expose the parathyroid glands, inferior thyroid artery and RLN (Fig. 7.12). The recurrent nerve usually passes behind the inferior thyroid artery (in 80 % of patients), but occasionally it lies anterior to it (in 15–20 % of patients), or it can pass between the branches of the inferior thyroid artery. It is best found by careful dissection in close proximity to and below the artery. Commonly, the nerves can be palpated before they are seen by running a finger transversely across the trachea below the level of the inferior thyroid artery. Moreover, in operations employing the intraoperative nerve monitoring (IONM) system, the nerves can be localized before visual identification by using a nerve mapping technique (Fig. 7.13). The nerve can then be traced upward, and its position in relation to the thyroid can be determined (Fig. 7.14). Parathyroid glands that lie on the thyroid surface can be mobilized with their vascular supply and preserved *in situ*. The lower parathyroid gland is usually anterior to the RLN and caudal to the inferior thyroid artery. The upper parathyroid gland is usually in a more posterior position behind the thyroid gland, and posterior and medial to the RLN. The trachea is exposed once the inferior thyroid veins are ligated. Further dissection is carried out in a cephalic direction with preservation of the parathyroid glands and RLN. Modern energy-based devices for tissue dissection and haemostasis can be used during thyroidectomy, but care must be taken to avoid thermal damage to the RLN as well as to the parathyroid

Fig. 7.10 Division of the individual branches of the superior pole vessels helps to preserve the superior branch of the external laryngeal nerve

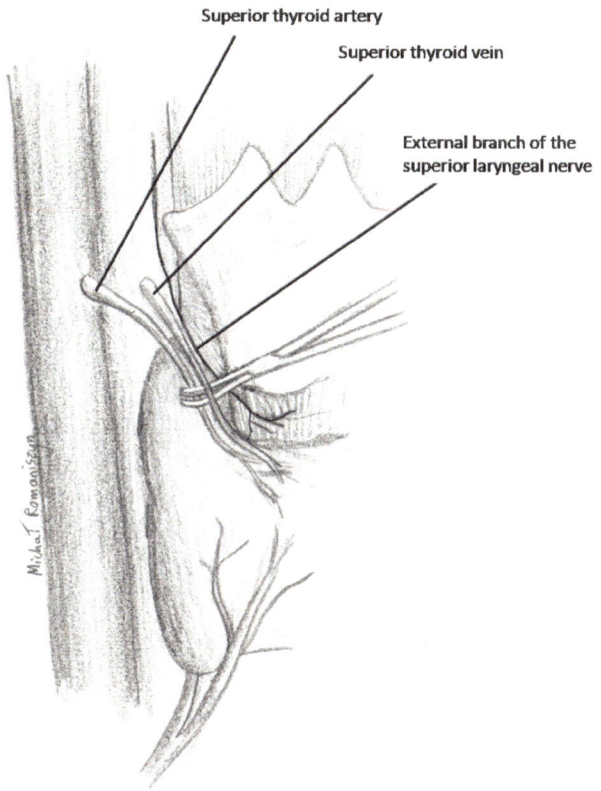

Superior thyroid artery

Superior thyroid vein

External branch of the superior laryngeal nerve

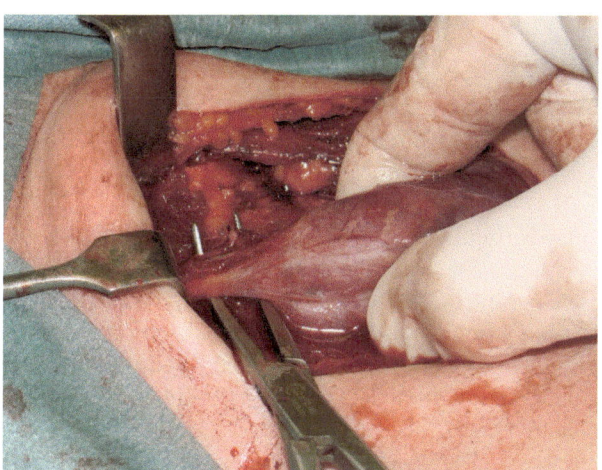

Fig. 7.11 Dissection of the individual branches of the superior thyroid pole vessels

Fig. 7.12 Recurrent
laryngeal nerve and its
relationship to
parathyroid glands and
ligament of Berry

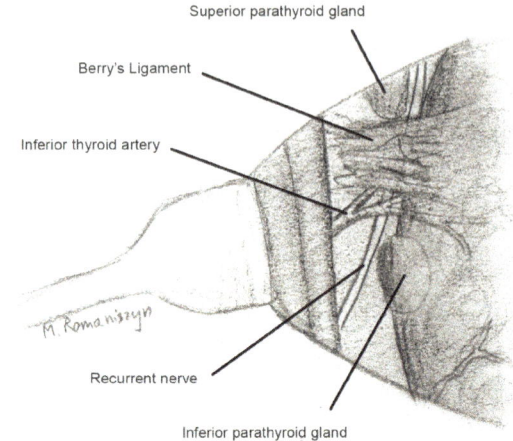

Superior parathyroid gland

Berry's Ligament

Inferior thyroid artery

Recurrent nerve

Inferior parathyroid gland

Fig. 7.13 Intraoperative
recurrent laryngeal nerve
mapping with bipolar
neural monitoring probe
allows for nerve
identification before its
visualization

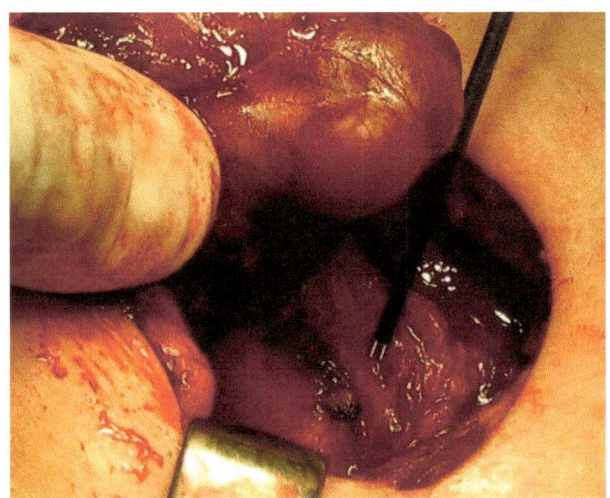

glands (Fig. 7.15). At the upper portion of the dissection, the RLN often lies on the
thyroid at the site of the ligament of Berry just before the nerve enters the posterome-
dial portion of the cricothyroid muscle. In this area the nerve is particularly vulnerable
to injury (for details *see* later in this section). Once the recurrent nerve is dissected free
from the thyroid gland and the Berry ligament is divided, the thyroid can be quickly
dissected free from the tracheal wall (Fig. 7.16). Near the midline, one should look for
the pyramidal lobe (if not dissected before), which should be dissected and included
in the surgical specimen. If a total thyroidectomy is intended, the isthmus should not
be divided and the contralateral thyroid lobe dissection performed in the same manner
as described above for the lobectomy to allow for *en bloc* thyroidectomy (Fig. 7.17).
If central compartment lymph node clearance (level VI) is planned, this should also be

Fig. 7.14 The right recurrent laryngeal nerve and parathyroid glands are preserved *in situ*

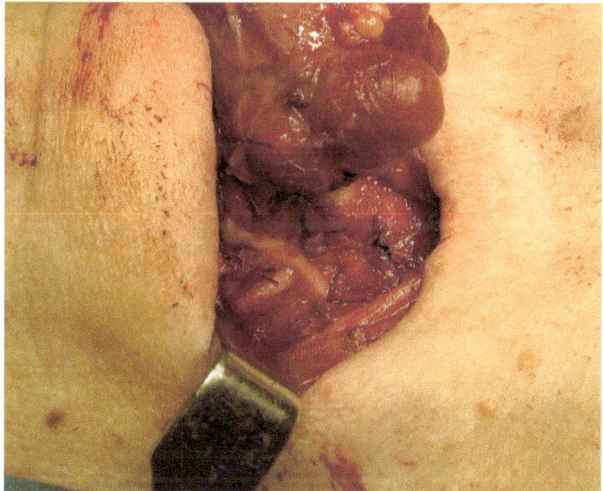

Fig. 7.15 Harmonic FOCUS dissecting shears device during thyroidectomy

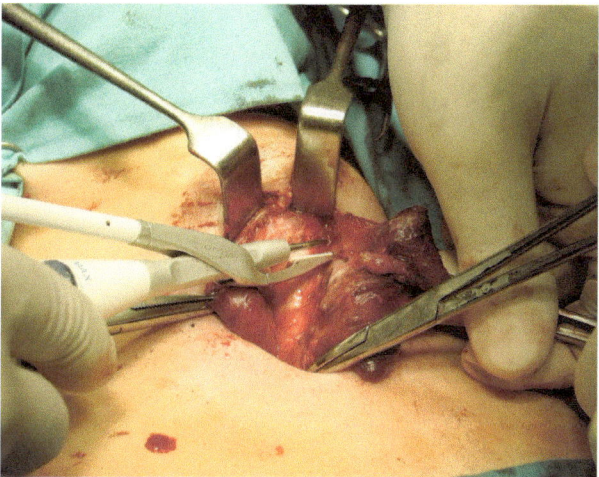

done as an *en bloc* dissection together with the entire thyroid gland (details below). The wound is then irrigated with warm saline and suction drains are placed. Wound closure is done in layers, with the sternothyroid and sternohyoid muscles reapproximated in the midline and the platysma sutured. The skin is closed with a running intracutaneous stitch, Steri-Strips™ (3 M HealthCare, Germany) or skin glue.

Central Compartment Lymph Node Dissection

Lymph node compartments separated into levels are shown in Fig. 7.18. The central compartment of the neck is a common site of local metastasis for papillary thyroid

Fig. 7.16 Final view of the operative field at the end of right hemithyroidectomy

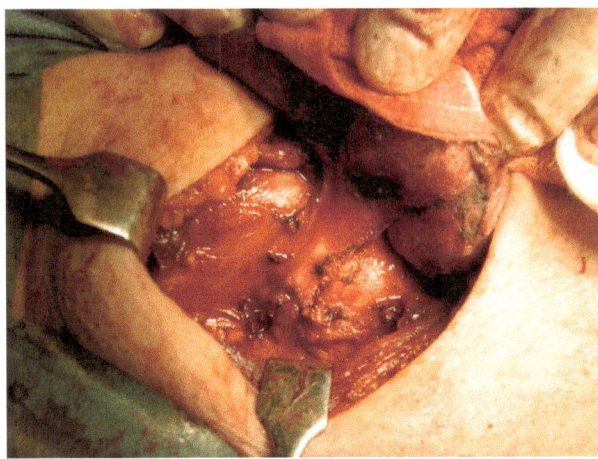

Fig. 7.17 Surgical specimen following *en bloc* total thyroidectomy (the superior pole of the left thyroid lobe containing the tumour is marked with a ligature for proper identification during pathological examination)

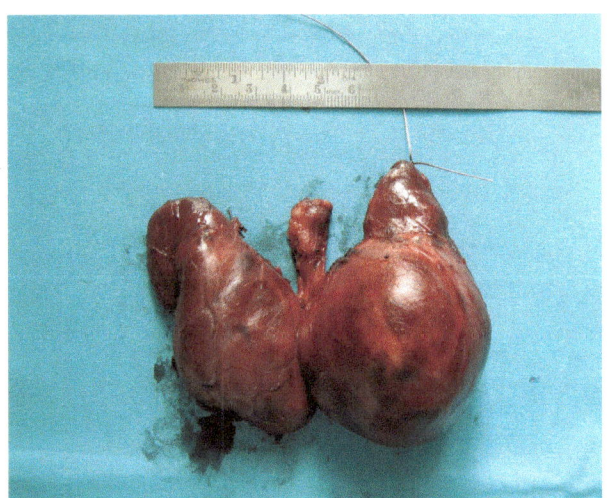

carcinoma (PTC). Therefore, for any surgeon who manages thyroid cancer patients, it is important to master knowledge of the surgical techniques employed during a central compartment neck dissection.

Systematic compartment-oriented central lymph node dissection may decrease the recurrence of PTC and probably improves disease-specific survival. Some data suggest a survival benefit with the addition of a prophylactic dissection to the thyroidectomy. The addition of compartment-oriented central lymph node dissection to total thyroidectomy can significantly reduce the levels of serum Tg and increase the rates of athyroglobulinaemia. However, there may be a higher rate of permanent hypoparathyroidism and unintentional permanent nerve injury when compartment-oriented central lymph node dissection is performed with total

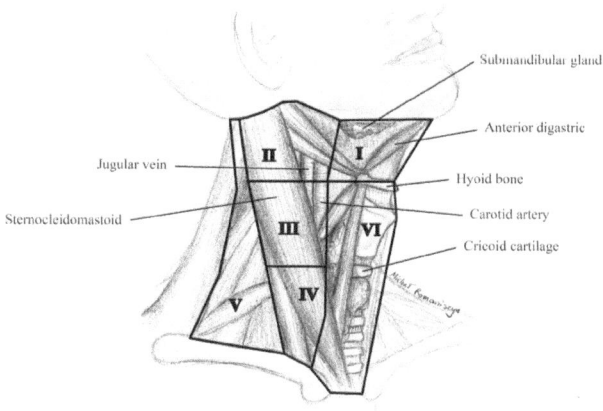

Fig. 7.18 Lymph node compartments separated into levels. Level VI contains the thyroid gland, and the adjacent nodes bordered superiorly by the hyoid bone, inferiorly by the innominate (brachiocephalic) artery, and laterally on each side by the carotid sheaths. The level II, III and IV nodes are arrayed along the jugular veins on each side, bordered anteromedially by level VI and laterally by the posterior border of the sternocleidomastoid muscle. The level III nodes are bounded superiorly by the level of the hyoid bone, and inferiorly by the cricoid cartilage; levels II and IV are above and below level III, respectively. The level I node compartment includes the submental and submandibular nodes, above the hyoid bone, and anterior to the posterior edge of the submandibular gland. Finally, the level V nodes are in the posterior triangle, lateral to the lateral edge of the sternocleidomastoid muscle. The inferior extent of level VI is defined as the suprasternal notch. Many authors also include the pretracheal and paratracheal superior mediastinal lymph nodes above the level of the innominate artery (sometimes referred to as level VII) in central neck dissection

thyroidectomy than total thyroidectomy alone. On the other hand, reoperation in the central neck compartment for recurrent PTC may increase the risk of hypoparathyroidism and unintentional nerve injury when compared with total thyroidectomy with or without compartment-oriented central lymph node dissection, supporting a more aggressive initial operation. Thus, standardization of the surgical approach to the central compartment is required in order to minimize morbidity and ensure comprehensive removal of all lymph nodes when indicated, which can reduce the need for reoperative dissections.

With regard to neck dissection, the term 'prophylactic' or 'elective' denotes removal of lymph nodes that are deemed normal pre- or intraoperatively by palpation and/or imaging studies. 'Therapeutic' or 'selective' dissection denotes removal of lymph nodes that possibly contain metastatic disease on the basis of palpation or imaging studies. 'Systematic' dissection refers to *en bloc* dissection of the anatomical neck compartments (which is recommended), as opposed to 'berry picking' of suspicious lymph nodes (which is not recommended).

The author prefers to perform a bilateral level VI lymph node dissection for PTC at the time of thyroidectomy for known PTC, using the technique previously described by the Delbridge group. The prelaryngeal lymph node, sitting directly anterior to the cricothyroid membrane between the cricothyroid muscles, is dissected at the time of mobilization of the thyroid pyramid and isthmus. Thyroidectomy is then completed using the technique described earlier. Once the gland is removed, attention is turned to the remaining level VI lymph nodes in the paratracheal and pretracheal spaces. The field is inspected to identify any macroscopic disease before dissection. Lateral dissection margins are defined using diathermy and surgical clips. The fibrofatty tissue in the midline is incised to expose the trachea down to the level of the brachiocephalic vessels inferiorly, and the medial border of the carotid artery is dissected down to the prevertebral fascia. The superior limit of dissection is at the level of the cricoid cartilage. The plane on the RLN is developed using a right-angled forceps, and a combination of surgical clips and sharp dissection. The nerve is freed from the fibrofatty tissue of the paratracheal space, allowing for lateral retraction of the RLN away from the level VI lymph nodes. Care is taken to preserve the superior parathyroid on a vascularized pedicle; the inferior parathyroid gland is typically devascularized and removed for autotransplantation by a slice technique, as described below. The envelope of tissue containing the level VI lymph nodes are then retracted medially and excised *en bloc* using a combination of diathermy and surgical clips to free it from the prevertebral fascia, oesophagus and trachea. The thymus is transected at the level of the brachiocephalic vessels and the specimen removed. The final surgical field should be clear of all fibrofatty and lymphatic tissue.

Methods of Laryngeal Nerve Preservation

Routine identification of the RLN is now part of treatment recommendations and is regarded as the gold standard of care in thyroid surgery.

The RLN crosses the inferior thyroid artery or its terminal branches at the level of the junction of the lower and the middle third of the thyroid lobe. The left RLN ascends at the depth of the TE groove or just lateral to it at the lower pole of the thyroid. Usually, it crosses deep to the inferior thyroid artery, sometimes between the terminal branches of the inferior thyroid artery—seldom superficially. The right RLN courses more obliquely, being caudally somewhat more lateral in position. It rarely crosses deep to the artery, usually between its terminal branches. In fact, the nerve is particularly prone to injury at the level of the inferior thyroid artery and in due course at the level of Berry ligament. Peripheral ligation of the branches of the inferior thyroid artery close to the thyroid capsule is the best way to preserve the nerve as well as the parathyroid glands. The RLN may be mistaken for a branch of the artery, particularly for the inferior laryngeal artery. The nerve is less regular, rounded and elastic than the artery. A small, red, tortuous vessel—the *vasa nervorum*—can be noticed on it. However, during traction when the nerve is under tension, this small vessel is barely visible. The nerve rarely bifurcates below the inferior thyroid artery, but the closer the entry into the larynx, the higher the chance of encountering a ramified nerve; this approaches 30 % at the level of the Berry ligament. Thus, the safest way to visualize the RLN is to search for it below the artery and, when identified, follow its course upward. Each extralaryngeal branch of the RLN should be preserved. At the two upper tracheal rings the nerve is embedded in the posterior portion of Berry ligament. This ligament extends posteriorly behind the RNL and loosely attaches the thyroid to the oesophagus. At the level of Berry ligament, the inferior laryngeal artery is located just posterior to the RLN and often gives off a small branch that crosses the nerve to enter the thyroid gland. Therefore, if there is any bleeding in this area, first the nerve needs to be identified before clamping the inferior laryngeal artery to avoid injury to the nerve. Moreover, medial traction of the thyroid lobe should be as gentle as possible in this area to avoid nerve paresis caused by pressure of the posterior fibres of Berry ligament on the nerve against the lateral aspect of the trachea. Instead, it is preferable to retract the lobe upward after complete dissection of its lower pole. This manoeuvre helps to follow the nerve until its entry into the larynx.

The non-recurrent inferior laryngeal nerve is a rare anatomical variant and is encountered in approximately 0.5 % of patients, almost always on the right side. The non-recurrent nerve arises as a vascular anomaly during embryonic development of the aortic arches and is associated with absence of the innominate artery and occurrence of an aberrant subclavian artery (*arteria lusoria*)—a condition that can be recognized preoperatively during Doppler ultrasound of the neck.

The following methods of RLN preservation can be considered:

- Visual nerve identification
- Use of magnifying glasses to facilitate nerve visualization
- Nerve palpation (against the trachea wall)
- Visual nerve identification with the aid of the IONM system.

Recent advances in thyroid surgery include IONM, which significantly aids visual identification of the RLN, allowing for nerve mapping even before its visualization, and provides the surgeon with a functional dimension previously not available with visual identification alone. Recently, it was documented in a randomized controlled trial that IONM decreased the incidence of transient, but not permanent, RLN paresis after thyroidectomy compared with visualization alone. The prevalence of transient RLN paresis was 2.9 % lower in high-risk patients who had RLN monitoring (p=0.01) and 0.9 % in low-risk patients (p=0.25). Despite these promising observations, the IONM technique is currently used mostly in high-volume thyroid surgery centres and is still under clinical assessment. It is up to each surgeon to decide whether to use nerve monitoring as a routine adjunct to each thyroid operation or to reserve it for more challenging operations. A recently published questionnaire study aiming to estimate the patterns of use of IONM devices during thyroid surgery by otolaryngologists in the United States of America documented that the majority did not report regular usage of RLN monitoring in their practices (only 28.6 % of responders admitted to using this device regularly). Surgical background and training, more than surgical volume, significantly influenced the use of IONM. However, it is also important to stress that RLN monitoring allows for nerve function documentation before and after thyroid resection (by printing the electromyographic signal of evoked potentials), which is of great importance in an increasing number of litigations.

Monitoring in the following three discrete modes of application may be considered:

1. *Identification ('neural mapping') of the RLN.* The nerve is mapped out in the paratracheal region through stimulation and then visually identified through directed dissection provided by the neural mapping. Multiple studies suggest IONM is associated with a rate of nerve identification of between 98 and 100 %.
2. *Aid in dissection.* Once the nerve is identified, additional intermittent stimulation of adjacent non-neural tissue against the nerve can help in tracing the nerve and all its branches through the dissected field in a way that is analogous to the use of intermittent facial nerve stimulation, as one dissects the facial nerve during parotidectomy.
3. *Prognostication of postoperative neural function and lesion site identification.* This has great significance in preventing bilateral vocal cord paralysis, given the frequent bilateral nature of the typical thyroid procedure. Prognostic statistics vary due to a number of factors but electrical testing of the nerve represents a significant improvement in accuracy of prognostic neural function when compared with the currently available test of visual inspection of the nerve.

The author personally believes that the aid of IONM nowadays plays an ever-increasing role in the surgical technique, thus paving the way for IONM-guided thyroid surgery.

During thyroidectomy, attempts should be made to preserve the external branch of the superior laryngeal nerves by ligation of the superior thyroid vessels at the capsule of the gland. It is also reasonable to first dissect the superior thyroid vessels away from the nerve by opening up a space between the cricothyroid muscle and the upper pole of the thyroid, and then divide the vessels as low as possible on the surface of the thyroid gland.

External laryngeal nerve injury has an associated morbidity, particularly in voice-quality changes (loss of vocal cords' tension makes it impossible to phonate with high-pitched voice sounds). Injury rates may be higher than for RLN damage, as it is usually overlooked at postoperative laryngoscopy.

Techniques for Preserving the Parathyroid Glands

The parathyroid glands should be identified and preserved whenever possible. Meticulous dissection and preservation *in situ* of all the parathyroid glands encountered during thyroidectomy has been accepted as routine clinical practice for many years. However, attempts at preserving a functioning parathyroid gland with a long pedicle are destined to fail in many cases, as it infarcts later because of thrombosis of the tenuous vascular supply, or as a result of oedema and swelling of the gland within its dissected capsule. If the vascular supply of preserved parathyroid gland/s is compromised, the gland/s should be excised and reimplanted into muscle. In such situations, as well as in cases of inadvertent removal of the parathyroid gland found on inspection of the thyroid capsule after resection, parathyroid autotransplantation is the only valid alternative that has been reported to reduce the incidence of permanent hypoparathyroidism.

Prior to any autotransplantation of the parathyroid gland, it is vital to send a small piece for frozen section to confirm that the autotransplanted tissue is truly a parathyroid gland and not a lymph node or metastatic thyroid cancer. Most thyroid surgeons employ the standard technique of parathyroid autotransplantation described by Wells et al. In this technique, the parathyroid tissue is placed in saline at 4 °C soon after excision. After cooling for 30 min, the gland is sliced into 1 mm slices (generally 10–20 pieces) and inserted into individual muscle pockets of the ipsilateral sternocleidomastoid muscle. The incisions are closed with nonabsorbable sutures. Use of many individual muscle pockets for parathyroid slices instead of only one or two pockets reduces the risk of graft insufficiency in case a haematoma forms around the transplanted tissue and results in avascular necrosis. As an alternative to Wells technique, parathyroid autotransplantation can be done using the parathyroid tissue injection technique, which is preferred by some surgeons. To minimize the risk of permanent hypoparathyroidism to almost zero, it also has been suggested to perform routinely elective parathyroid autotransplantation of at least one gland in all patients undergoing thyroid surgery. In spite of the fact that such a strategy effectively prevents persistent hypoparathyroidism, it increases significantly the incidence of transient hypoparathyroidism requiring prolonged calcium medication for 12–18 weeks. To avoid this drawback of elective parathyroid autotransplantation, a tailored approach to parathyroid reimplantation, based on the result of an iPTH assay, might be beneficial for patients, resulting in a zero risk of permanent hypoparathyroidism and a markedly reduced incidence of transient hypocalcaemia. An intraoperative iPTH level that is within the reference range soon after total thyroidectomy indicates that at least two parathyroid glands are functioning well and the risk of permanent hypoparathyroidism may be considered low. On the other hand, a drop in the iPTH plasma level below the lower limit of the reference range (<10 ng/L) should be regarded as a permanent deficiency of at least three parathyroid glands, until proven otherwise, which means a high risk of permanent hypoparathyroidism. It is important to remember that lymph node dissection in the central compartment (level VI) is associated with an increased risk of postoperative hypoparathyroidism. Thus, all high-risk patients would benefit most from parathyroid reimplantation, while in low-risk patients, parathyroid autotransplantation could be abandoned in order to avoid increasing the incidence of transient hypoparathyroidism. Regardless of which approach to parathyroid autotransplantation is used, whether it be liberal routine reimplantation or more conservative selective, and on the basis of clinical judgement supported by the result of intraoperative iPTH assay, a combination of both preservation of the parathyroid glands *in situ* and by autotransplantation is essential in modern thyroid surgery, thereby reducing the risk of permanent hypoparathyroidism after total thyroidectomy to almost zero.

Common Mistakes

1. The incision should not be placed too low in the neck as it makes it very difficult to safely expose the vessels of the superior poles of the thyroid gland and endangers the external branch of the superior laryngeal nerve.
2. If the thyroid tumour is large, the sternohyoid and sternothyroid muscles should be transected without hesitation.
3. Gentle traction of the thyroid lobe should be used instead of traction with clamps.
4. The RLN should be first identified at the level of its crossing with the inferior thyroid artery before any of the branches of the artery are ligated.
5. The common trunk of the inferior thyroid artery should never be ligated because if this manoeuvre is performed bilaterally, it involves a serious risk of permanent hypoparathyroidism. Instead, the capsular ligation technique should be used.
6. In case of a large substernal goitre the superior pole of the thyroid lobe should be dissected first.
7. The thyroid specimen should be inspected carefully soon after thyroidectomy and any parathyroid glands removed inadvertently should be re-implanted into one of the sternocleidomastoid muscles.
8. When central compartment lymph node clearance (level VI) is performed, great care must be taken to not injure the RLNs and not remove the inferior parathyroid glands.

Commentary

Frederick L. Greene

This chapter on the surgical treatment of thyroid disease is both extremely well written and complete with regard to our current approach to well-differentiated thyroid cancer. The management of this disease has certainly changed over the past three to four decades, during which time we have learned more about the biology of this cancer and the fact that microscopic sites of tumour may develop synchronously throughout the gland. Differentiated thyroid cancer, especially papillary tumours, may be multicentric in a majority of patients and, therefore, bilateral lobar extirpation is certainly appropriate. Because of this aggressive approach to well-differentiated thyroid tumour, the technical issues, and especially the important anatomical considerations to avoid injury to the RLN and parathyroid glands, have become especially cogent.

Referencing data from the National Cancer Database, which has been developed by the American College of Surgeons Commission on Cancer in conjunction with the American Cancer Society, the author appropriately notes that total surgical ablation of the thyroid gland has increased over the past 20 years and now represents ~90 % of thyroidectomies for well-differentiated thyroid neoplasms. The experience of the surgeon, as well as the environment in which the surgeon works, seem to have an effect on the aggressiveness of the approach to thyroid cancer, and will obviously have an effect on the overall outcome. Management guidelines have also been developed by the American Thyroid Association and other groups, indicating that a more aggressive approach to well-differentiated thyroid cancer is appropriate.

The technique of total thyroidectomy is of paramount importance and needs to be taught to every young surgeon who does thyroid resections. Injury to the parathyroid glands and RLNs needs to be minimized and, happily, this has occurred in more modern databases of thyroid surgery. Specialization in head and neck surgery, and especially thyroid surgery, has shown that repetitive operations and a higher volume of procedures tend to reduce the likelihood of anatomical injury. Appropriate credentialing and privileging must be mandatory in order to create an environment in which safe thyroid surgery can be performed. This approach will also include appropriate knowledge of the lymph node compartments in the neck, which frequently harbour well-differentiated thyroid carcinoma. Because the central compartment of the neck is a common site of local metastasis, the appropriate technique of dissecting this area is mandatory. The author comments on the technique of performing a bilateral level VI lymph node dissection for papillary thyroid carcinoma and this is certainly becoming more popular worldwide.

Appropriate thyroid surgery begins with good planning by both the surgeon and the operative team. Full disclosure to the patient regarding the potential complications and benefits of the procedure are mandatory. Only then can safe surgical ablation for thyroid cancer be performed.

Suggested Reading

Barczyński M, Konturek A, Cichoń S. Randomized controlled trial of visualization versus neuro-monitoring of recurrent laryngeal nerves during thyroidectomy. *Br J Surg* 2009;**96:**240–6.

Bilimoria K, Bentram D, Linn JG, *et al*. Utilization of total thyroidectomy for papillary thyroid cancer in the United States. *Surgery* 2007;**142:**906–13.

Bilimoria KY, Bentrem DJ, Ko CY, *et al*. Extent of surgery affects survival for papillary thyroid cancer. *Ann Surg* 2007;**246:**375–81.

Cooper DS, Doherty GM, Haugen BR, *et al*. Revised American Thyroid Association management guidelines for patients with thyroid nodules and differentiated thyroid cancer. *Thyroid* 2009;**19:**1167–214.

Cady B, Rossi R. An expanded view of risk-group definition in differentiated thyroid carcinoma. *Surgery* 1988;**104:**947–53.

Grodski S, Lachlan C, Sywak M, *et al*. Routine level VI lymph node dissection for papillary thyroid cancer: Surgical technique. *ANZ J Surg* 2007;**77:**203–8.

Haigh PI, Urbach DR, Rotstein LE. AMES prognostic index and extent of thyroidectomy for well-differentiated thyroid cancer in the United States. *Surgery* 2004;**136:**609–16.

Hundahl SA, Fleming ID, Fremgen AM, *et al*. A National Cancer Data Base report on 53,856 cases of thyroid carcinoma treated in the U.S., 1985–1995. *Cancer* 1998;**83:**2638–48.

Hay ID, Thompson GB, Grant CS, *et al*. Papillary thyroid carcinoma managed at the Mayo Clinic during six decades (1940–1999): Temporal trends in initial therapy and long-term outcome in 2444 consecutively treated patients. *World J Surg* 2002;**26:**879–85.

Sosa JA, Bowman HM, Tielsch JM, *et al*. The importance of surgeon experience for clinical and economic outcomes for thyroidectomy. *Ann Surg* 1998;**228:**320–30.

Minimally Invasive Approach to the Thyroid

8

Istvan Gal

This chapter presents current trends in minimally invasive procedures for thyroid cancers. Minimally invasive video-assisted thyroidectomy is discussed in detail.

Introduction

Thyroidectomy, one of the most common operations worldwide, has a low morbidity rate if performed by skilled surgical teams. However, conventional thyroidectomy requires a transverse cervical incision (Kocher incision) that leaves a visible scar on the anterior surface of the neck. The application of minimally invasive techniques for thyroid surgery was motivated primarily by an attempt to improve the cosmetic results of this operation. The aesthetic point of view is particularly important for young women, as they constitute a large part of the patients affected by thyroid disease. Initial reports of minimally invasive procedures for removal of thyroid nodules were published between 1997 and 1999. In the past decade, several techniques for video-assisted and purely endoscopic thyroidectomy have been described. Video-assisted approaches generally use a small incision in the neck region. Pure endoscopic techniques use an axillary, or breast, or an axillo-bilateral-breast approach. In these techniques, incisions for trocar placement are situated far from the neck. The operative field is exposed using carbon dioxide insufflation. The advantage of these procedures is that no visible scar is seen in the neck region. It should be emphasized that these procedures are technically demanding and require a surgical team skilled in both endocrine and endoscopic surgery. This is particularly true for endoscopic thyroidectomy by the axillary or breast approach. Another

I. Gal
Department of Surgery, Telki International Private Hospital,
Telki, Hungary
e-mail: galistv@gmail.com

© The Author(s) 2012
F.L. Greene, A.L. Komorowski (eds.), *Clinical Approach to Well-differentiated Thyroid Cancers*, Head and Neck Cancer Clinics,
DOI 10.1007/978-81-322-2568-3_8

concern is the invasiveness of the procedures. The concept of surgical invasiveness cannot be limited to the length or site of the skin incision. It must be extended to all structures dissected during the procedure. Therefore, minimally invasive thyroidectomy should be properly defined as an operation through a short (1.5–3 cm) incision that permits direct access to the thyroid, resulting in a focused dissection. In addition, the type of anaesthesia, the duration of the operation, postoperative pain, complications and success rates, as well as long-term outcomes should also be taken into account when assessing surgical invasiveness.

Postoperative recovery after conventional thyroidectomy is prompt. Findings have shown that the minimally invasive video-assisted thyroidectomy (MIVAT), as proposed by Paolo Miccoli from the University of Pisa, Italy, and which has become popular in recent years, has some advantages over conventional surgery in terms of cosmetic result, postoperative distress and postoperative recovery. The procedure permits direct access to the thyroid through a 1.5–2 cm central skin incision above the sternal notch through which a total thyroidectomy can be achieved.

Oncological Aspects

Surgery is the foremost, and generally sole, effective treatment for well-differentiated thyroid cancers, disregarding iodine-concentrating tumours that can be treated in some cases by radio-iodine therapy. Because the growth patterns of these tumours vary, the extent of dissection should be tailored to the respective tumour entity, especially for less aggressive tumours. However, the extent of thyroidectomy for well-differentiated thyroid cancer remains controverversial. According to a recently published, comprehensive national study from the USA, the short-term outcomes for unilateral and complete thyroidectomy are significantly different; complications are more frequent after total thyroidectomy than after a unilateral procedure (15 % versus 6 %; $p \leq 0.0001$). Therefore, the decision about whether or not to perform total thyroidectomy can be influenced by concerns regarding the risk of such devastating complications as bilateral recurrent laryngeal nerve (RLN) palsy or permanent hypoparathyroidism, neither of which is a concern when unilateral lobectomy is performed. On the other hand, compelling data exist that show an improvement in survival and recurrence rate after more extensive thyroid surgery when compared with limited resection. If all patients with papillary thyroid carcinoma (PTC) underwent total thyroidectomy, the estimated improvement in long-term survival would be ~2 %. Although the differences in outcomes seem small when expressed as a percentage, the number of patients affected would be relatively large. According to data from the literature, commonly adopted staging systems for well-differentiated thyroid cancer can be applied not only for PTC, but also specifically for follicular thyroid carcinoma (FTC) too. Risk factors and risk group analysis are important for the management of patients with FTCs, although currently published therapeutic guidelines call for total thyroidectomy followed by radioactive iodine (^{131}I) ablation for all patients with FTC. The distinction of FTCs into minimally invasive and invasive carcinomas is based on the extent of invasiveness rather than on vascular invasion. It

Table 8.1   Criteria for minimally invasive video-assisted thyroidectomy

Presence of a nodule not >35 mm in maximum diameter
Thyroid volume ≤25 ml – evaluated by ultrasound
Absence of thyroiditis in biochemical or ultrasound studies
Cytological and clinical evidence of benign disease, and/or low-risk papillary, minimally invasive follicular carcinomas. (Diagnosis of minimally invasive follicular carcinoma can be made either on the basis of capsular invasion alone, vascular invasion alone, or the presence of both types of invasions. A pathological distinction between low-grade minimally invasive [encapsulated] and widely invasive follicular thyroid carcinoma, as suggested by WHO, is valid for prognosis and has been adopted in guiding treatment of follicular thyroid carcinoma – *see also* Chap. 2.)
Absence of enlarged lymph nodes in the neck on ultrasound
No previous neck surgery or irradiation

is important to identify patients with low-risk follicular carcinoma to offer them more conservative treatment. Hemithyroidectomy can be considered as adequate treatment for patients with minimally invasive cancer after histological confirmation, whereas total thyroidectomy followed by adjuvant I^{131} therapy should be reserved for patients with invasive cancer on the basis of histomorphological criteria, or for high-risk patients identified by using commonly adopted staging systems.

Minimally invasive video-assisted and complete endoscopic thyroidectomy were introduced in clinical practice to treat small thyroid nodules (Table 8.1). The effectiveness of MIVAT for surgical treatment of well-differentiated thyroid cancer is still debatable. However, the literature from the past few years confirms that the MIVAT procedure is a safe and valid option for patients with low-risk, well-differentiated thyroid cancer. In a study by Miccoli et al., 171 patients operated on with low- and intermediate-risk PTC by the MIVAT technique were compared with 50 patients operated on by conventional thyroidectomy. After a mean follow up of 3.6 ± 1.5 years (range 1–8 years; median 5 years), both groups showed comparable outcomes, and cumulative ^{131}I activity was administered to achieve curative status. Lombardi et al. published a series of 271 patients with PTC operated by the MIVAT procedure. In each case, either a total thyroidectomy or a lobectomy was performed, followed by completion thyroidectomy. Using the same approach, a central neck node removal was done in 102 patients. Postoperative complications included transient recurrent nerve palsies (5 patients), transient hypocalcaemia (59 patients), permanent hypoparathyroidism (3 patients), and postoperative haematoma (1 patient). Follow-up evaluations were completed for 231 patients. Mean postoperative serum thyroglobulin after levothyroxin withdrawal was 5.5 ng/ml. No residual thyroid tissue was evident in any of the patients on postoperative ultrasonography. Mean postoperative ^{131}I uptake was 2.1 %. Only 1 patient developed a lateral neck recurrence. Other data support the opinion that the completeness of the operative resection achieved with video-assisted thyroidectomy seems comparable with that reported for conventional surgery. However, MIVAT can be applied only to a minority (10–15 %) of cases, i.e. only for the treatment of low-risk, well-differentiated carcinoma. Factors that influence the best operative approach include tumour size, histology, the presence of enlarged lymph nodes, and evidence of locoregional invasion. According to the AJCC/TNM staging system, patients aged <45 years with stage I disease, or patients aged ≥45 with stage I or stage II disease may be candidates for the procedure. On the basis of the AGES (age, grade, extent, size) scoring system, patients with ≤3.99 points may be selected for MIVAT. On the basis of the AMES (age, metastasis, extent, size) scoring system, patients at low risk may be selected for MIVAT (for more information on the AGES and AMES systems, *see* Chap. 5).

Surgical Procedure

Recommended Set for MIVAT

- Forward-oblique telescope 30°, diameter 5 mm, length 29 cm, autoclavable
- Miccoli suction dissector with cut-off hole, with stylet, blunt, length 21 cm
- Miccoli elevator, 2 mm wide, blunt, length 19 cm (two pieces recommended)
- Miccoli vessels suspender hook, malleable, length 21 cm
- Miccoli tissue retractor, length 16 cm, double-ended, 35×10 and 21×10 mm (two pieces recommended)
- Bellucci scissors, working length 8 cm, 8 mm blade
- Grasping forceps, working length 15 cm, rough serrated
- Reddick–Olsen grasping forceps, rotating, size 3 mm, length 20 cm, heavy, with connector pin for unipolar coagulation
- Scissors, rotating, size 3 mm, length 20 cm, serrated, curved, conical, with connector pin for unipolar coagulation, double action jaws
- Bipolar coagulating forceps
- Clip applier, diameter 5 or 10 mm, rotating, for small-size titanium and/or plastic vascular clips
- Ultrasonically activated shears (optional).

Description of the Procedure

Preparation of patients for the procedure is similar to that for conventional thyroid surgery. The patient, under general anaesthesia, is placed in the supine position with no hyperextension of the neck (Fig. 8.1). A 15–25 mm horizontal incision is given ~2 cm above the sternal notch. A simple method for determining an optimal incision (Fig. 8.2) has been reported by Gui-Zhou Xiao and Li Gao. Subcutaneous fat and the platysma are carefully dissected to avoid bleeding. The cervical linea alba is divided longitudinally for at least 3 cm. The strap muscles on the affected side are then gently retracted with a small conventional retractor; a second retractor is placed directly on the thyroid lobe, which is retracted medially and lifted up. The two small retractors maintain the operative space. A 30° 5 mm endoscope is inserted through the skin incision (Fig. 8.3). Dissection of the thyrotracheal groove is completed

Fig. 8.1 Position of the patient for MIVAT (note no neck hyperextension as compared to Fig. 7.1)

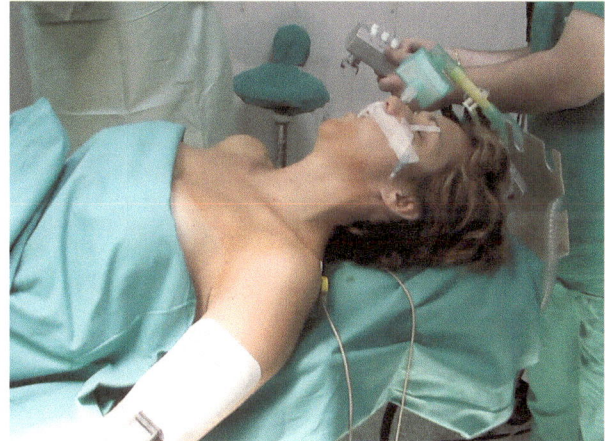

Fig. 8.2 A simple method for determining an optimal incision (based on Xiao and Gao 2008). *1* Midpoint of sternal notch, *2* midpoint of thyroid notch, *3* midpoint of mental region, *4* this point is marked 2 cm above point *1* in the midline, Points *5* and *6* equally distant from point *4* are marked symmetrically in the perpendicular line. The distance between the points is the planned incision (length 1.5–2.5 cm)

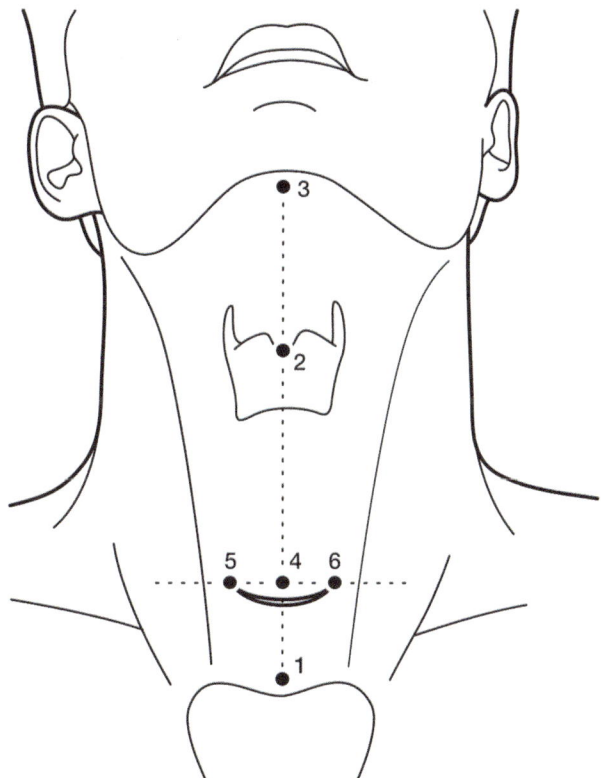

under endoscopic vision (Figs. 8.4 and 8.5) using the above-mentioned instruments, i.e. atraumatic spatulas, spatula-shaped aspirator, dissector and scissors.

Avoiding electrocautery (either bipolar or monopolar) is particulary important when the laryngeal nerves are not yet exposed. Haemostasis is hence achieved by

Fig. 8.3 Introducing the endoscope into the operative field

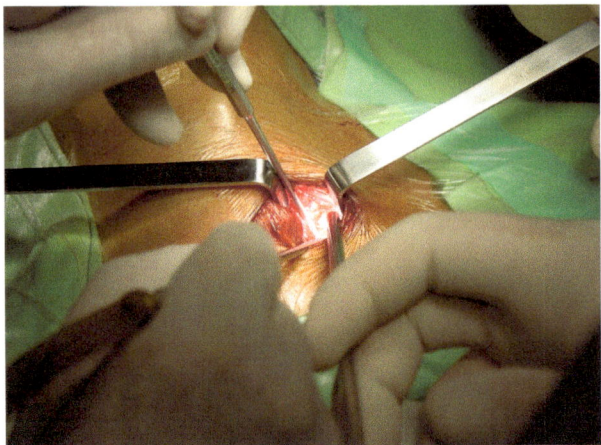

Fig. 8.4 Dissection of the thyrotracheal groove under endoscopic visualization

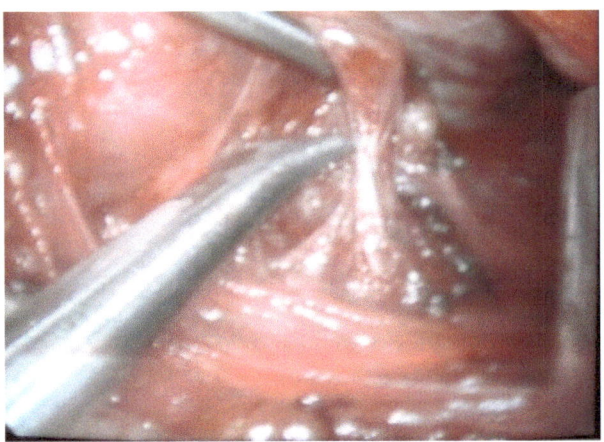

means of small (3 mm) conventional vascular clips or ultrasonically activated shears. The first vessel to be ligated is the middle vein, if present, or the small veins between the jugular vein and the thyroid capsule. The upper pedicle is then exposed. The thyroid lobe is retracted downward by the retractor. The spatula is used to separate the larynx from the vessels and to retract them laterally. The vessels are then selectively ligated by vascular clips and cut. The external branch of the superior laryngeal nerve can be easily identified during most procedures once the different components of the upper pedicle have been prepared. The inferior vessels are also clipped and cut, exposing the anterolateral side of the trachea.

After retracting medially and lifting up the thyroid lobe, the fascia can be opened by a gentle spatula retraction. The RLN generally lies in the thyrotracheal groove (Fig. 8.6), behind the Zuckerkandl tubercle. The parathyroid glands can be visualized easily because of endoscopic magnification. During dissection, haemostasis is achieved by clips or ultrasonic shears. In this way, the RLN and the parathyroid glands are dissected and freed from the thyroid.

Fig. 8.5 Continued dissection of the thyrotracheal groove under endoscopic visualization

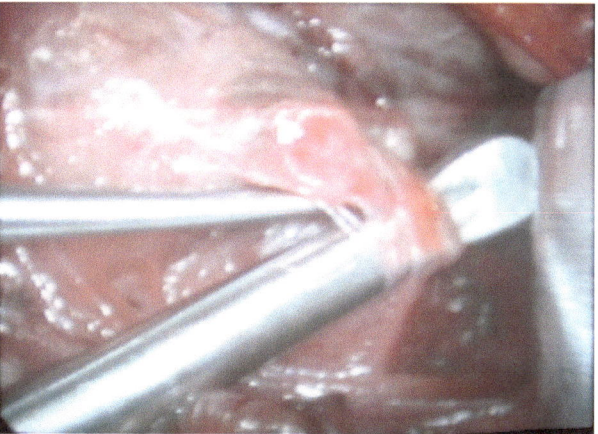

Fig. 8.6 The recurrent laryngeal nerve (*dotted*) after removal of the involved lobe of the thyroid gland

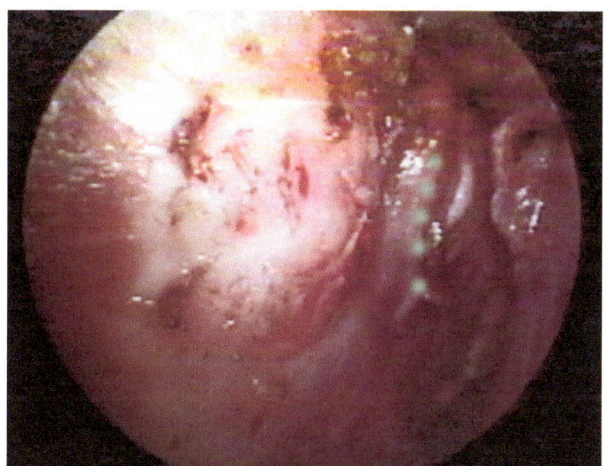

After removing the endoscope and the retractors, the surgeon carefully pulls out the upper portion of the gland using conventional forceps. Gentle traction over the lobe allows the gland to be completely pulled out. The operation is now conducted as in open surgery under direct vision (Fig. 8.7). It is very important to check the RLN once again to avoid injury to it before the final steps. The isthmus is then dissected from the trachea and divided. In case of total thyroidectomy, the operation is continued on the opposite side in the same manner. After completely exposing the trachea, the lobe and/or the complete thyroid gland are finally removed by the conventional open technique (Fig. 8.8). A drainage is usually not necessary but optional, depending on the surgeon's decision. The linea alba and platysma are sutured with absorbable sutures and the wound is closed either by a subcuticular running suture or with skin sealant (Fig. 8.9).

Fig. 8.7 Resection of the removed thyroid lobe by ultrasonically activated shears

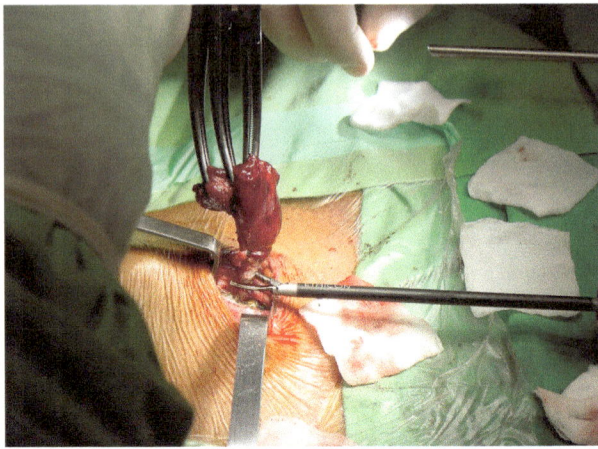

Fig. 8.8 Subtotally resected thyroid gland removed after MIVAT

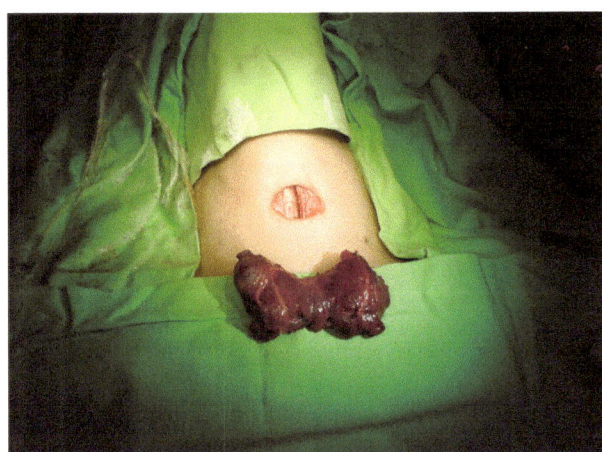

Complications

According to the literature, in terms of complications MIVAT is comparable with conventional thyroidectomy procedures. In a study by Miccoli et al. involving 1320 patients with benign and malignant thyroid lesions treated with MIVAT (lobectomy 421; total thyroidectomy 899), operative complications included transient unilateral RLN palsy in 35 cases (2.65 %) and definitive unilateral RLN palsy in 15 cases (1.13 %). Thirty-eight patients suffered transient hypoparathyroidism, which corresponds to 4.2 % of the total thyroidectomies performed, but only 2 patients had permanent hypoparathyroidism. Conversion to standard cervicotomy was required in 30 patients (2.2 %). Of a total of 521 patients, Lombardi et al. observed 9 (1.7 %) with transient RLN palsies, 73 (14 %) with transient hypocalcaemia, 3 (0.6 %) with definitive hypoparathyroidism, 1 (0.2 %) with postoperative haematoma, and 2 (0.4 %) with wound infections. Conversion was necessary in 6 patients (1.2 %)

Fig. 8.9 Closing the incision by a skin sealant

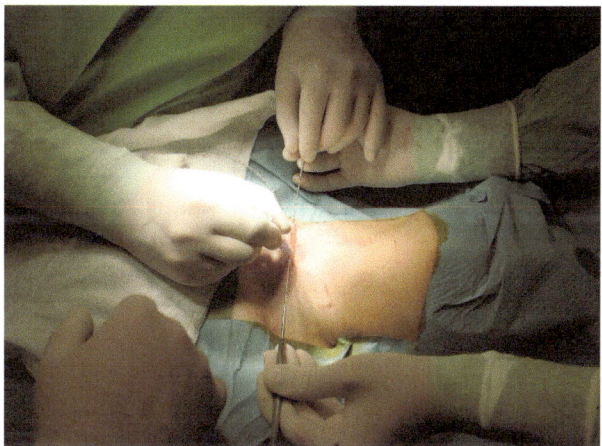

Fig. 8.10 The cosmetic result of MIVAT. Six months after surgery the scar is barely visible

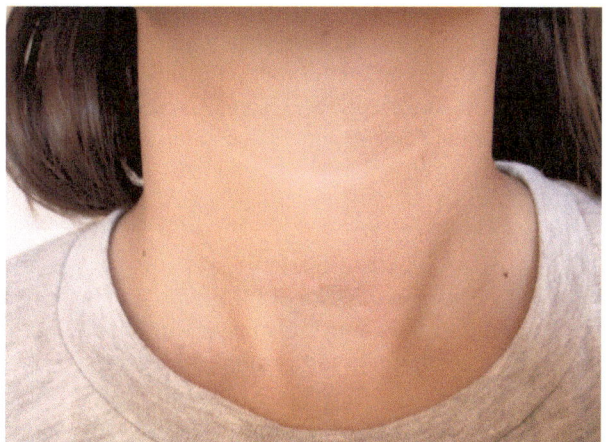

(difficult dissection in 1 patient, large nodule size in 3 and gross lymph node metastases in 2 patients).

Reported data confirm that MIVAT achieves the same clearance at the thyroid bed level and the same outcome as the conventional technique when dealing with 'low-risk', well-differentiated cancers. At the same time, a select group of patients can benefit from the advantages of this technique, which include lower postoperative pain, faster postoperative recovery and excellent cosmetic outcome (Fig. 8.10).

Future Perspectives

Neck surgery is one of the newest fields of application of minimally invasive surgery. The technique of MIVAT previously described and developed by Miccoli is the procedure that has become most popular. Limiting factors of this access include the 15–25 mm cervical incision and, consequently, the specimen size to be removed. Several other approaches (via the chest, axillary, breast or bilateral axillary breasts) are also in use. The development of cervical scarless thyroid surgery is a great step toward better cosmetic outcomes. However, with these techniques, the scars have moved from the neck region to other regions where they are still visible. Therefore, the next step seems to be natural orifice surgery. In general, the goals of minimally invasive thyroid surgery will be to fulfil the following criteria:

1. Respect surgical planes.
2. Access to the operative field should be close to the gland to achieve a minimally invasive procedure.
3. Leave no scar.
4. Minimize trauma.
5. The minimally invasive character of this approach and the optimal cosmetic result should not be reached at the expense of the patient's safety.

There is currently no procedure which fulfils all these requirements. However, in the author's opinion, when applied judiciously, minimally invasive thyroid surgery, as described above, offers advantages over conventional surgery and is an appropriate component of head and neck endocrine practice.

Common Mistake

The most common mistake of the minimally invasive access to the thyroid is incorrect selection of patients. This may result in a higher percentage of patients requiring conversion to the traditional open surgery.

Commentary

Pietro Iacconi and Gabriele Materazzi

This is an exhaustive chapter on recently developed minimally invasive techniques for thyroidectomy, and primarily describes MIVAT. The role and results of this technique for the treatment of thyroid carcinoma are correctly described and discussed in depth, both from the technical and oncological points of view.

To recapitulate the goals described by the author of the minimally invasive thyroid approach, the technique should encompass the following criteria: (i) Surgical planes should be respected; (ii) access to the operative field should be close to the gland; (iii) scar tissue should not remain; (iv) trauma should be minimized; and (v) results of the minimally invasive technique must not be achieved at the expense of the patient's safety.

On the whole, among the various recent minimally invasive/endoscopic approaches, MIVAT seems to represent the technique that most respects these criteria.

MIVAT was ideated and developed by Paolo Miccoli in Pisa in 1998, and from the very beginning of Miccoli's experience, inclusion criteria for selecting patients undergoing MIVAT were established. These inclusion criteria are limited to the number of patients that can benefit from this approach, but which ultimately result in the patient's safety, good postoperative recovery and excellent cosmetic outcome.

MIVAT can be performed in 10–15 % of thyroid cancer patients. Absolute contraindications include the following conditions: Thyroiditis, nodules >3 cm, cancers >2 cm, and cancers with the presence of lymph nodes metastases. In fact, if these contraindications are ignored, the cosmetic result and safety of the technique is compromised. Local implants after minimally invasive thyroidectomy have been reported; this could be related to morcelization of a large goitre, which undoubtedly does not represent a correct indication for MIVAT. Furthermore, the large volume of the thyroid obviously hampers safe dissection of important structures, such as the laryngeal nerves and parathyroids during the 'endoscopic' step of the procedure.

The majority of papers published on MIVAT report that no difference is seen in the complication rate between MIVAT and traditional thyroidectomy. However, these series (MIVAT versus conventional surgery) are, in fact, not statistically comparable; MIVAT series are constituted by selected patients, whereas the traditional thyroidectomy series usually range from small thyroid glands to large, intrathoracic or locally invasive carcinomas.

There is no doubt that MIVAT offers the following advantages:

- Magnification of the target by employing the endoscope; this allows optimal visualization of the superior and inferior laryngeal nerves and of the parathyroid glands.
- The possibility of exploring both sides with a small, unique, median incision
- Less pain because the patient does not need neck hyperextension
- An easy technique for general surgeons to learn, because it reproduces traditional thyroidectomy
- The operation can be converted easily into a conventional open approach.

Small, non-aggressive tumours can be safely treated by MIVAT. However, the question arises of whether is it possible always to make this diagnosis preoperatively. All the important series on MIVAT show that a great number of tumours (of the less aggressive variety) are treated with this approach and that the same survival rate is achieved as with traditional thyroidectomy. One criticism that could be raised is that the median length of follow up (5 years) reported in the largest series is not enough to exclude recurrence when dealing with this type of neoplasia. The literature documents that differentiated thyroid cancer has a long survival with a low recurrence rate, independent of the type of surgical treatment. Nevertheless, as reported by Miccoli et al., despite the fact that a longer follow up is necessary before drawing any final conclusions, the first 5 years from the diagnosis of papillary carcinoma and initial treatment are those with the highest risk of recurrence.

Temporary laryngeal nerve palsy rate after MIVAT appears to be higher than that after traditional thyroidectomy. This is not due to an excessive traction on the nerve during the extraction of the lobe, if the nerve has been properly dissected during the endoscopic phase, but might be caused by improper utilization of energy devices, such as ultrasonic scissors employed during the operation. It is well known that the minimal distance of the active blade must be >5 mm. When necessary, a vascular clip is preferable when dealing with small vessels close to the nerve, in order to achieve total removal of thyroid tissue, instead of leaving a remnant in order to 'preserve' the nerve.

All authors underline better cosmetic results with MIVAT. Of course, a blind trial is impossible.

The traction on the skin makes contusion of the verges mandatory, thus causing the premise for a suboptimal scar. The decision is to perform a smaller but a more 'worked out' incision or longer incision (comprising contused margins).

One of the advantages of MIVAT is the reduction of postoperative pain; it is expected that both the absence of neck hyperextension and more limited dissection concur in this aim. A prospective, randomized study was designed to demonstrate objectively that MIVAT minimizes postoperative pain. TGF-β serum levels immediately after surgery seem to correlate with levels of pain, confirming that reduced postoperative distress is an objective of MIVAT. This result confirms the results of studies based only on subjective pain evaluations (Miccoli et al. *Surg Endosc* 2010).

As for the disadvantages of the technique, the following must be considered:

• There must be three surgeons—one for the camera, one for retractors and the operator.
• The learning curve needs at least 30 procedures.

I agree with the author that the most common mistake of MIVAT is an incorrect selection of patients.

Can we consider minimally invasive procedures by the transaxillary or the breast approach to the thyroid—or even TOVAT (transoral video-assisted thyroidectomy)? All these procedures look cumbersome; some need carbon dioxide insufflation, similar to one of the first attempts by Gagner, with a prolonged stay in the recovery room. All this effort is made to avoid a scar in the neck by paying the price of a demanding (and possibly risky) procedure.

MIVAT is a technique in some ways equivalent to single port access in abdominal laparoscopic surgery; a minimally invasive approach becoming increasingly popular. Some new instruments will probably be employed (or modified) for thyroid procedures.

About the future evolution of this field, it is hoped that evolution of robotic arms will broaden the indications for MIVAT.

Finally, one more application for MIVAT is the sentinel node study procedure with the preliminary injection in the tumour and localization of the sentinel node.

Suggested Reading

Benhidjeb T, Wilhelm T, Harlaar J, *et al.* Natural orifice surgery on thyroid gland: Totally transoral video-assisted thyroidectomy (TOVAT): Report of first experimental results of a new surgical method. *Surg Endosc* 2009;**23:**1119–20.

Del Rio P, Sommaruga L, Pisani P, *et al.* Minimally invasive video-assisted thyroidectomy in differentiated thyroid cancer: A 1-year follow-up. *Surg Laparosc Endosc Percutan Tech* 2009;**19:**290–2.

Huscher CS, Recher A, Napolitano G, *et al.* Endoscopic right thyroid lobectomy. *Surg Endosc* 1997;**11:**877.

Lombardi CP, Raffaelli M, de Crea C, *et al.* Report on 8 years of experience with video-assisted thyroidectomy for papillary thyroid carcinoma. *Surgery* 2007;**142:**944–51.

Lombardi CP, Raffaelli M, Princi P, *et al.* Video-assisted thyroidectomy: Report of a 7-year experience in Rome. *Langenbecks Arch Surg* 2006;**391:**174–7.

Miccoli P, Berti P, Conte M, *et al.* Minimally invasive surgery for small thyroid nodules: Preliminary report. *J Endocrinol Invest* 1999;**22:**849–51.

Miccoli P, Berti P, Raffaelli M, *et al.* Comparison between minimally invasive video-assisted thyroidectomy and conventional thyroidectomy: A prospective randomized study. *Surgery* 2001;**130:**1039–43.

Miccoli P, Pinchera A, Materazzi G, *et al.* Surgical treatment of low- and intermediate risk papillary thyroid cancer with minimally invasive video-assisted thyroidectomy. *J Clin Endocrinol Metab* 2009;**94:**1618–22.

Miccoli P, Berti P, Ambrosini CE. Perspectives and lessons learned after decade of minimally invasive video-assisted thyroidectomy. *ORL J Otorhinolaryngol Relat Spec* 2008;**70:**282–6.

Miccoli P, Rago R, Massi M, et al. Standard versus video-assisted thyroidectomy: objective postoperative pain evaluation. *Surg Endosc* 2010;24(10):2415–17. doi:10.1007/s00464-010-0964-7.

Wada N, Hasegawa S, Masudo Y, *et al.* Clinical outcome by AMES risk definition in Japanese differentiated thyroid carcinoma patients. *Asian J Surg* 2007;**30:**102–7.

Xiao GZ, Gao L. A simple method for determining an optimal incision for minimally invasive video-assisted thyroidectomy. *Surg Endosc* 2008;**22:**2100–101.

Zerey M, Prabhu AS, Newcomb WL, *et al.* Short-term outcomes after unilateral versus complete thyroidectomy for malignancy: A national perspective. *Am Surg* 2009;**75:**20–4.

Management of Advanced Thyroid Cancer: Local Recurrence and Neck Dissections

Ettienne J. Myburgh

The focus of this chapter is on the management of locally advanced disease, lymphadenectomy and treatment of recurrent disease in patients with well-differentiated thyroid cancers.

Introduction

Although well-differentiated thyroid carcinoma (WDTC) accounts for only 2 % of cancers and is responsible for only 0.5 % of cancer-related deaths, between 8 and 23 % of patients develop local recurrence. Autopsy studies have found that 15 % of patients with WDTC will have invasion outside the thyroid capsule. In spite of this, follicular and papillary carcinomas have a good long-term prognosis. Only a small group of patients do poorly, and several risk classifications have been described to identify high-risk patients. Invasion of structures outside the thyroid has been consistently shown to be an independent predictor for mortality and local recurrence.

Initial Evaluation of the Patient with Loco-Regionally Advanced Disease

The following clinical signs of soft tissue involvement should be sought:

- A large fixed mass
- Local or referred pain

E.J. Myburgh
Department of Surgery, Panorama Medi-Clinic and Head, Neck and Breast Unit,
Tygerberg Academic Hospital, Cape Town, South Africa
e-mail: surgery@mweb.co.za

© The Author(s) 2012
F.L. Greene, A.L. Komorowski (eds.), *Clinical Approach to Well-differentiated Thyroid Cancers*, Head and Neck Cancer Clinics,
DOI 10.1007/978-81-322-2568-3_9

- Vocal fatigue or hoarseness
- Chronic non-productive cough, late-onset 'asthma' or stridor
- Haemoptysis
- Dysphagia.

Special Investigations

Fine-needle aspiration is routinely used to assess suspected thyroid masses or nodes, and can confirm the diagnosis in the majority of cases. Ultrasound evaluation can give valuable information about non-palpable pathological neck nodes, involvement of vascular structures, and an indication of local extension. Indirect laryngoscopy should be utilized liberally to evaluate vocal cord function. The recurrent laryngeal nerve (RLN) should be assessed for damage during previous surgery or for infiltration by a tumour. Dysphagia and haemoptysis should be evaluated endoscopically to identify mucosal or submucosal tumour involvement of the trachea or oesophagus.

^{123}I whole-body scintigraphy can indicate iodine absorption by tumour tissue as well as the presence of residual thyroid tissue and metastatic lesions. The use of single-photon emission computerized tomography (SPECT) to localize non-palpable disease is very helpful.

CT and magnetic resonance imaging (MRI) are valuable for evaluating the regional anatomy. High-resolution spiral CT is generally utilized because of its widespread availability, lower cost and fast image acquisition. It gives superior assessment of cartilaginous invasion, and software manipulation of images aids pre-operative visualization. However, intravenous contrast administration may interfere with the uptake of iodine isotopes for up to 6 weeks. MRI has the advantage of not using iodine contrast. The assessment of soft tissue involvement is excellent but it takes longer to acquire images, and image manipulation is limited.

Metastatic work-up should be routinely done in patients with extrathyroidal infiltration or recurrent disease.

Chest X-ray is usually inadequate to assess pulmonary and mediastinal involvement. CT evaluation is superior and can be done during evaluation of the neck. The use of positron-emission tomography (PET)/CT is valuable in patients whose thyroglobulin levels are raised and ^{123}I-imaging is negative. The presence of high false-positivity should be interpreted in conjunction with results from other imaging modalities.

For a more detailed description of imaging possibilities in thyroid cancer, *see* Chap. 4.

Management of the Neck Nodes

Lymph node metastases are present in an average of 60 % of patients with papillary carcinoma; lymphadenopathy may be the presenting complaint in ~15 % of patients. In spite of this, the long-term survival remains good. Current opinion is that lymph node involvement increases the risk for recurrence and mortality although purely micrometastic disease does not necessarily equate with a worse prognosis, especially in young patients. Surgical removal of the lymph nodes remains the mainstay of treatment. Radioactive ^{131}I and/or external beam radiotherapy do not compensate for macroscopic disease left behind during surgery. Complete clearance of all macroscopic disease is paramount in achieving a cure.

Central Neck Dissection

The central compartment is defined superiorly by the hyoid bone, inferiorly by the brachiocephalic vessels, laterally by the carotid sheath and posteriorly by the prevertebral fascia. It contains the prelaryngeal (Delphian), pretracheal, paratracheal, retro-oesophagal and retropharyngeal nodes, and is generally referred to as level VI (*see* Fig. 7.18).

Dissection of the central compartment (level VI) might be applicable in the absence of gross lymphadenopathy, but this remains controversial. This is the region where most local recurrences occur, leading to significant morbidity caused by involvement of the surrounding structures. The aim is to reduce the recurrence rate and gain a survival advantage. Several large series (e.g. SEER [Surveillance, Epidemiology and End Results database]) have shown a survival benefit with prophylactic central lymph node dissection (CLND), but this has not been confirmed and the importance of occult micrometastatic disease remains unclear. The main risk of adding CLND to total thyroidectomy is the possibility of hypoparathyroidism and RLN paralysis. The decision to perform CLND should be based on the risk of recurrence and mortality in the individual patient, and carefully weighed against the potential morbidity. As most thyroid operations are not performed in specialized centres, the decision may be dependent on the available local expertise.

Current Indications for Central Lymph Node Dissection

- Clinical or radiological evidence of pathological nodes in level VI
- High-risk papillary carcinoma with signs of extrathyroidal spread
- Relative indications include men aged >50 years and large primary tumours.

The primary aim is to remove all macroscopic disease; the extent of the dissection for microscopic disease should be balanced against the risk to the parathyroids and RLN.

Lateral Neck Dissection

In the past, the concept of 'berry picking' (i.e. removing single, grossly involved nodes only), was widely practised. This has been shown to have a very high rate of recurrence (100 % after berry picking versus 9 % after selective lymphadenectomy) and as such is no longer appropriate. Evidence is scant that prophylactic lateral neck dissection adds any benefit to the management of WDTC.

Therapeutic dissection has been shown to reduce recurrence and improve survival. There are conflicting guidelines with regard to the extent of the dissection. Many authors advise dissecting only levels III and IV, citing a very low incidence of nodal metastases in the other levels. A recent publication by Caron et al. reported that only 3 % of the patients developed nodal recurrence in either level I or V nodes. Positive nodes in level I only occurred in association with significant disease in level II. When only levels III and IV were dissected, 21 % of the patients required further dissection of level II. Of some concern is the fact that in spite of level II dissection, 19 % of the patients developed recurrence in level II.

On the basis of this it would be sensible to perform levels III and IV dissection if limited disease is found in level IV. If nodes are present in level III, then level II should be included in the dissection. Level I should be added only if gross disease is present in level II.

In most cases, when extranodal disease is not present, the sterno-cleidomastoid muscle, spinal accessory nerve and jugular vein can be spared. Any sign of tumour involvement of any of these structures would necessitate *en bloc* resection of these.

Management of Locally Advanced Disease

Extended Resection of Locally Advanced Disease

Strap Muscles

The sternothyroid, sternohyoid and omohyoid muscles are frequently involved (57 %) when local invasion is present but this does not seem to influence prognosis, although systemic metastases are more common. Resection of these muscles adds little to morbidity and clear surgical margins should be obtained with *en bloc* resection. Resection of the whole muscle is not necessary.

Recurrent Laryngeal Nerve

In 50 % of cases with histologically confirmed infiltration, vocal cord paralysis was not found preoperatively, and in 67 % no vocal change was reported preoperatively. Bilateral vocal cord paralysis should be avoided at all costs. The contralateral, uninvolved nerve must be assessed with care to avoid this complication and a subsequent tracheostomy. If both nerves are involved by the tumour, every effort should be made to preserve one functioning nerve. If microscopic disease is left on the nerve while attempting to preserve it, it does not affect the prognosis adversely.

In patients with no preoperative vocal cord function, the nerve can be resected if it is found to be invaded by the tumour intraoperatively.

If the vocal cord was functioning preoperatively, attempts should be made to preserve the nerve when it is not involved grossly by the tumour. Often, the nerve will be found running over the surface of the tumour. Under these circumstances, the nerve may be dissected free with the knowledge that microscopic residual tumour will remain, for which radioactive iodine or external beam radiotherapy should be considered postoperatively. If preservation of the nerve necessitates leaving macroscopic residual disease, the nerve should be resected *en bloc*.

The resected nerve can be repaired, as both nerve repair and medialization give similar long-term results. Either option is superior to no treatment of the paralysed cord. Medialization is performed most commonly and can improve voice quality in the majority of patients. Although it can be done at the time of the initial surgery, this procedure is generally performed postoperatively. It should be considered early on in the postoperative period in elderly patients, as they have less capacity to compensate and are at greater risk for aspiration.

Laryngotracheal Infiltration

The most common cause of death in thyroid cancer is tracheal obstruction. Between 7 and 10 % of thyroid cancers may invade the trachea. The perichondrium is not an effective barrier to tumour invasion, allowing early invasion of the cartilage and into the submucosa.

Several surgical options have been described to deal with laryngotracheal involvement. Shave procedures aim at removing all macroscopic tumour from the airway while avoiding resection. Partial resections aim to resect the tumour fully while maintaining full function and limiting the need for extensive reconstruction and later complications. Full resections aim to radically remove the tumour, along with the affected larynx or trachea.

Regardless of the technique used, recurrence and mortality rates are high if complete tumour clearance is not achieved.

Shaving Procedures

Complete resection using a shave procedure is the most suitable option if the tumour does not invade the cartilage. Invasion into the mucosa or submucosa is clearly a contraindication. Early cartilagous involvement might still be amenable to shaving although the morbidity and mortality of resection of the larynx should be weighed against the likely risk of recurrence and death.

Laryngeal Resection

Involvement of the larynx is rare and, as such, the choice of procedure should be individualized. Several partial laryngeal resections have been described. Fifty per cent of the laryngeal cartilage can be resected while the mucosa is preserved with no need for reconstruction. Thirty per cent of the cricoid cartilage can also be resected. When a larger resection is necessary, a reconstructive procedure will be required. Several innovative techniques have been described for immediate, delayed or staged reconstructions.

Total laryngectomy is seldom necessary but should be considered for transmural involvement, haemorrhage and loss of laryngeal function.

Tracheal Resection

Tracheal invasion can occur through the cartilage rings or the soft tissue in between the tracheal rings; it is inclined to spread circumferentially rather than vertically.

Several techniques for partial resection can be utilized, including window resection, wedge resection and partial resection with periosteal or muscle flaps. Window resection of the trachea is appropriate if no more than one ring is involved and infiltration is limited to the cartilage. It is simple to perform. Deeper infiltration or more extensive involvement requires segmental resection of the trachea with primary anastomosis. Care should be taken to avoid damage to the RLNs and vascular supply to the trachea originating from the inferior thyroid artery and running laterally. Resection of 5–6 cm can be performed without mobilization of the larynx and carina but this may vary from patient to patient. Longer resections are possible with release of the larynx. With division of the thyrohyoid muscles and thyrohyoid membrane, ~2 cm of length can be obtained. One should avoid entering the pharynx during this mobilization. For more mobility the suprahyoid muscles may also be divided. Techniques for mobilization of the pulmonary hilum to gain more length for extended resections have been described by Grillo et al. in 1964.

Anastomotic complications can be expected in 9 % of patients. Factors that adversely influence outcome are reoperation, diabetes, resections of ≥4 cm, laryngotracheal resection, age <17 years, and need for a tracheostomy preoperatively.

The tracheal anastomoses should be performed with interrupted 3-0 or 4-0 prolene sutures. Knots should be secured extraluminally Closure starts in the middle of the posterior wall and proceeds laterally until the anterior wall is closed. In most cases the endotracheal tube can be left in place, but alternatively a reinforced endotracheal tube may be placed into the distal trachea and connected to the anaesthetic machine while the orotracheal tube is retracted into the proximal laryngotrachea. Once the posterior wall has been secured, the distal tracheal tube may be removed with advancement of the orotracheal tube beyond the anastomoses, allowing further closure of the anastomosis. On completion, an airtight seal of the anastomosis can be confirmed by flooding the operative field with saline and requesting the anaesthesthetist to perform a Valsalva manoeuvre with a deflated cuff. A tracheostomy should be avoided as far as possible, as it increases the risk for anastomotic complications.

After skin closure, the submental skin is sutured to the presternal skin with a loose nylon suture to maintain neck flexion for 2–3 weeks. Patients are generally extubated after 24 h.

Oesophageal Involvement

The oesophagus may be infiltrated by the primary tumour or by paratracheal nodes with extranodal spread. In most cases, the oesophageal muscle is involved and the mucosa spared. This allows resection of the involved muscle while sparing the mucosa. As long as the mucosa is intact, no reconstruction is needed. In cases of deeper infiltration, partial resection can be achieved with primary, layered closure. Previous radiation, circumferential involvement, or extensive involvement requires segmental resection of the oesophagus. If a short segment of healthy oesophagus is resected, primary closure may be feasible. If a tension-free anastomosis cannot be achieved, two options are available, i.e. transhiatal resection of the oesophagus with gastric pull-up or interposition of the colon or jejunum. If microsurgical expertise is available, a free jejunal transfer to the resected segment could be considered. Other methods have been described and local expertise and policy will dictate the procedure of choice. The placement of a gastrostomy or ileostomy tube for postoperative feeding should be considered.

Vascular Infiltration

Only 38 cases of venous infiltration by thyroid carcinoma have been reported in the literature. It is a rare occurrence and has a very poor prognosis. The jugular vein can be resected in most cases, but saphenous vein interposition might be required in selected cases of reoperation.

Carotid artery involvement is rare and encasement of the artery rather than invasion is usually the case. Reconstruction can be done with prosthetic material or the saphenous vein. A muscle flap should be considered to cover the arterial reconstruction, especially when radiotherapy is considered or concomitant tracheal resection is performed.

Management of Recurrent Disease

A single recurrence does not seem to influence the ultimate prognosis but repeated recurrences are associated with a significant risk for future recurrence and death. The main risk factors for mortality and repeated recurrence are age >45 years, extrathyroidal spread, vascular invasion, stage III/IV disease, MACIS score of >6 (*see* Chap. 5), and a recurrence developing within 12 months of surgery. These factors probably identify tumours with aggressive biological behaviour rather than inadequate initial therapy. However, 30 % of these patients can be rendered disease-free with repeated procedures.

The aim of treatment is to resect all disease fully. Recurrences could be in the thyroid bed, where microscopic tumour is left behind after surgery, or in one or more nodes.

In cases in which previous lymph node dissection and/or total thyroidectomy have not been performed, a CLND and completion thyroidectomy should be performed at the time of resecting the recurrence. Neck nodes are managed as stated in the section on neck dissection.

If a recurrence occurs within the previously dissected neck or thyroid bed, the aim is complete excision of the recurrence only. Scarring due to previous surgery and radiation is an additional challenge, but complete resection can usually be accomplished with low morbidity. Several techniques are available to aid identification of the tumour within the surrounding scar tissue. Only recurrences of >10 mm should be considered for resection. Careful preoperative planning is essential and good imaging is indispensible. Intraoperative ultrasound can be very helpful in planning incisions and the surgical approach. The utilization of hook-wire localization has been reported and can be helpful if the recurrence is not located close to the major vascular structures or too superficially. Preoperative injection with blue dye or carbon can help localize recurrence within the scar tissue.

Summary

Although patients with WDTC have a good prognosis, a minority will develop more advanced disease. Complete resection of the entire tumour provides a good long-term cure to most patients. If high-risk patients can be identified preoperatively appropriate surgical planning can achieve effective surgical clearance with minimal morbidity and good long-term results.

Commentary

Tahar Benhidjeb

This chapter on the management of advanced thyroid cancer is concise and well written. It contains all the information required for daily practice.

The management of advanced thyroid cancer represents a surgical challenge because of the complex anatomy of the neck region and the gland's close topographic relationship to adjacent organs. The optimal goal is to improve overall survival (or at least progression-free survival). This can be achieved by an operation that encompasses radical removal of the entire tumour and invaded structures. Accurate preoperative staging to determine the resectability and assess the extent of resection is a *conditio sine qua non* in surgical planning. The approach presented in this chapter corresponds to the way our group treats patients with advanced thyroid cancer.

Suggested Reading

Carling T, Long WD 3rd, Udelsman R. Controversy surrounding the role for routine central lymph node dissection for differentiated thyroid cancer. *Curr Opin Oncol* 2010;**22**:30–4.

Carty SE, Cooper DS, Doherty GM. Consensus statement on the terminology and classification of central neck dissection for thyroid cancer. *Thyroid* 2009;**19**:1153–8.

Holler T, Theriault J, Payne RJ, *et al.* Prognostic factors in patients with multiple recurrences of well-differentiated thyroid carcinoma. *J Oncol* 2009;**2009**:650340.

Patel KN, Shaha AR. Locally advanced thyroid cancer. *Curr Opin Otolaryngol Head Neck Surg* 2005;**13**:112–16.

Price DL, Wong RJ, Randolph GW. Invasive thyroid cancer: Management of the trachea and oesophagus. *Otolaryngol Clin North Am* 2008;**41**:1155–68, ix–x.

Rotstein L. The role of lymphadenectomy in the management of papillary carcinoma of the thyroid. *J Surg Oncol* 2009;**99**:186–8.

Shah JP, Patel SG. Thyroid and parathyroid glands. In Shah JS (ed). *Head and neck surgery and oncology*. 3rd ed. New York: Mosby; 2003:424–8.

Sippel RS, Chen H. Controversies in the surgical management of newly diagnosed and recurrent/residual thyroid cancer. *Thyroid* 2009;**19**:1373–80.

Stanisław Kłęk

This chapter covers nutritional problems in thyroid cancer patients. The specific nutritional issues related to thyroid cancer, as well as to surgery, radiotherapy, chemotherapy and palliative care are discussed.

Introduction

Nutritional issues in thyroid cancer can be analysed from two points of view: (i) General (thyroid function in unaffected and in altered nutritional status, potentially influencing further carcinogenesis); and (ii) oncological (nutritional approach to oncological treatment). Unlike cancers in some other organs, nutritional problems associated with thyroid cancer are of utmost importance.

General Considerations

In most cases, particularly in the European setting, thyroid diseases are irreversibly connected with either an excess or deficiency of iodine in the diet. Iodine deficiency results, among other complications, in irreversible mental and neurological retardation, reproductive complications, hypothyroidism and goitre. The latter is the most obvious manifestation of iodine deficiency, essentially because it is one of the earliest and easiest to notice. More important is that iodine deficiency or the administration of goitrogens, often demonstrated by the presence of goitre, may lead to thyroid tumours. In the presence of a carcinogen or irradiation to the thyroid, high yields of

S. Kłęk
Department of General Surgery, 1st Chair of General Surgery, Jagiellonian
University Medical College and Nutrimed Medical Corporation, Krakow, Poland
e-mail: klek@poczta.onet.pl

© The Author(s) 2012
F.L. Greene, A.L. Komorowski (eds.), *Clinical Approach to Well-differentiated
Thyroid Cancers*, Head and Neck Cancer Clinics,
DOI 10.1007/978-81-322-2568-3_10

101

malignant thyroid tumours may be obtained. Goitrogens or iodine deficiency lead to a lowering of thyroid hormone levels in the blood with a consequent homeostatic increase in the levels of thyroid-stimulating hormone (TSH). If continuous, this leads to the formation of thyroid adenomas.

A normal diet contains a harmless quantity of progoitrine and its activator, but in some situations, such as an undifferentiated diet (e.g. vegetarian or vegan), the amount of these substances may expose the individual to the risk of developing a goitre.

As thyroid cancer (a follicular subtype in particular) is more common in areas where goitre and iodine deficiency are endemic, it has been hypothesized that dietary factors, especially iodine intake, may influence the risk of this cancer. Studies in the Polish population showed a direct relationship between iodine deficiency and the occurrence of goitre. In the early 1980s, the Polish government ceased the iodization of table salt and the frequency of goitre increased rapidly; the reverse process was observed when the iodization was reinstated in the 1990s.

Nutritional factors other than iodine deficiency can also be instrumental in causing goitre. A study of diet and thyroid cancer conducted in Sweden and Norway showed that people living in areas of endemic goitre in Sweden had an elevated risk of developing thyroid cancer, especially women. Among persons who had ever lived in such areas, high consumption of cruciferous vegetables was associated with an increased risk. Regardless of the area of residence, high consumption of butter and cheese was associated with a significantly increased risk of thyroid cancer. The association with consumption of iodized salt in Norway showed a weak, inverse relationship. Among women, the regular use of vitamin A, C or E supplements was associated with a decreased risk.

On the other hand, an excess of iodine may result in hypothyroidism, autoimmune thyroid disease and papillary thyroid cancer (PTC). Some studies showed that the incidence of PTC increased proportionately with an increasing intake of iodine in the population, and that correcting the iodine deficiency shifts the ratio of follicular to PTC, in favour of the latter.

Malnutrition and Thyroid Cancer

Oncological patients suffer frequently from malnutrition; up to 80 % of patients diagnosed with malignant disease are at risk for malnutrition, which causes a higher incidence of postoperative complications, increased length of hospital stay and, consequently, higher costs of treatment.

It is unclear if thyroid function is decreased in malnutrition, because some studies showed an increase and others a decrease in thyroid function. Animal studies have confirmed that when an animal consumes less energy than required for maintenance, as occurs in malnutrition, energy might be conserved by a decrease in thyroid function and thermogenesis. These metabolic changes would serve to enhance survival potential when the diet is inadequate or the protein content of the diet is low. This suggests that in thyroid cancer patients, malnutrition results in an unfavourable clinical course not because of deterioration in hormonal activity, but because of a deteriorating function of the whole organism.

According to the European Society for Clinical Nutrition and Metabolism (ESPEN), the therapeutic goal for cancer patients is the improvement of function and outcome by taking the following steps:

- Preventing and treating undernutrition
- Enhancing anti-tumour treatment effects
- Reducing the adverse effects of anti-tumour therapies
- Improving the quality of life.

Nutrition and Surgical Approach

The subject of nutritional approach in cancer surgery was presented widely in the guidelines published by ESPEN in 2006. The most important points are presented below:

1. Preoperative fasting is unnecessary in most patients.

   Commentary: A study on enhanced recovery after surgery proved that in the absence of impaired motility, delayed gastric emptying or intestinal obstruction, and if there was no risk of aspiration, the patient could cease fluid intake just 2 h before the operation. Such a strategy was seen to result in a better prognosis (e.g. pain control, faster recovery, shorter hospital stay, etc.). Apart from the patient being allowed to drink fluids up to 2 h before anaesthesia, he or she can eat solid food up to 6 h before anaesthesia. Moreover, it is recommended that a preoperative carbohydrate-rich drink be administered to most surgical patients.

2. Patients with severe nutritional risk should be given nutritional support for 10–14 days before major surgery, even if the surgery has to be delayed. Severe nutritional risk refers to at least one of the following criteria: Weight loss of 10–15 % within 6 months, body mass index of <18.5 kg/m^2, Subjective Global Assessment Grade C, serum albumin of <30 g/L (with no evidence of liver or kidney dysfunction).

   Commentary: The routine use of parenteral nutrition, particularly hyperalimentation, led to an increased complications' ratio. Therefore, its use in all surgical patients is no longer recommended. On the other hand, the introduction of enteral nutrition, isocaloric feeding and restriction of parenteral nutrition enabled successful postoperative recovery. Preoperative nutritional support in malnourished patients helps to reduce postoperative complications and shortens the length of hospital stay.

   It is important to consider and start nutritional intervention (enteral route is the method of choice if it is not contraindicated) even in patients without obvious

Table 10.1 Indications for nutritional intervention in patients not suffering from malnutrition

Patients who are anticipated to be unable to eat for 7 days after surgery
Patients whose food intake after 7 days post-surgery will not be >60 % of protein and caloric requirements

malnutrition. Indications for nutritional intervention in such patients are summarized in Table 10.1. In patients who cannot meet their nutritional requirements by the enteral route, parenteral nutrition should be encouraged.

3. Use enteral nutrition peri-operatively, preferably with immunomodulating substrates (omega-3 fatty acids, arginine, nucleotides), irrespective of the nutritional risk of patients undergoing major neck surgery for cancer.

    Commentary: Although the real value of immunomodulatory nutrition in surgical patients has been questioned recently, doubts do not concern preoperative intervention in high-risk patients, such as those undergoing major head and neck surgery. These patients are likely to benefit from such treatment.

4. Consider placement of a percutaneous endoscopic tube (PEG) if long-term (>4 weeks) tube feeding is necessary, e.g. in severe head injury.

    Commentary: These recommendations should be considered particularly carefully in patients who need palliative care and in whom thyroid carcinoma threatens to obstruct the gastrointerstinal tract. PEG placement, mentioned above, should always be considered as the treatment of choice.

Non-surgical Oncology

The nutritional issues faced by patients with thyroid cancer can be associated with non-surgical methods, i.e. radiotherapy, chemotherapy, hormone therapy and palliative treatment. The European Society for Clinical Nutrition and Metabolism provides the following guidelines in such situations:

1. *General recommendations*
   - Nutritional assessment of cancer patients should be performed frequently and nutritional intervention initiated early when deficits are detected.
   - Reliable data of the effect of enteral nutrition on tumour growth is lacking. Such theoretical considerations should, therefore, not influence the decision to feed a cancer patient.

2. *Nutritional recommendations during radio- or radiochemotherapy*
   - Intensive dietary advice and oral nutritional supplements are advocated to increase dietary intake and to prevent therapy-associated weight loss and interruption of radiation therapy.
   - Routine enteral nutrition is not indicated during radiation therapy or chemotherapy.
   - Tube feeding can be delivered via either the transnasal or percutaneous routes, but because oral and oesophageal mucositis occur frequently, PEG is advised.

3. *Nutritional recommendations for incurable patients*
- Enteral nutrition should be administered to minimize weight loss, as long as the patient consents to it and the dying phase has not begun.
- When life is coming to an end, most patients require only minimal amounts of food and a little water to reduce thirst and hunger. Small amounts of fluid may also help to avoid states of confusion induced by dehydration.
- Pharmacological interventions should be recommended in addition to nutritional intervention in the presence of systemic inflammation in order to modulate the inflammatory response.
- In cachectic patients, steroids or progestins are recommended to enhance appetite, modulate metabolic derangements, and prevent impairment of the quality of life. The benefits of using steroids should be weighed against their adverse effects.

Special Nutritional Considerations in Thyroid Cancer

The special nutritional considerations for thyroid cancer patients include the recommendation of a hypophosphataemic diet in patients who have undergone surgery or radioactive iodine therapy and demonstrate signs of hypoparathyroidism, as well as the careful choice of diet in hyper- and hypothyroidism (the latter requires increased protein and water intake). Recently, some authors have observed that fluoride administration induces thyroid dysfunction; dietary calcium and the plasma protein level may influence this relationship and reverse it, but this has been observed only in animal models. Others have noted that ghrelin, the gastrointestinal hormone, inhibits thyroid cell proliferation in thyroid cell carcinoma. The real clinical value of these observations is uncertain and further studies are warranted.

Common Mistakes

Most surgeons disregard nutritional issues in thyroid cancer patients. Nutritional screening is performed occasionally; nutritional intervention is rare even in malnourished patients, and the majority of patients undergo unnecessary preoperative fasting. Most patients are not even informed about nutrition (dietary counselling) and the use of oral nutritional supplements during radio- or radiochemotherapy.

Commentary

Andrzej L. Komorowski

'Most surgeons disregard nutritional issues in thyroid cancer patients.' I think this phrase, which is true not only of surgeons, summarizes the essential message of this chapter. Our treatment decisions have to be based on facts. Whereas it is completely acceptable not to give any nutritional support to our patients, this decision has to be based on the evaluation of his/her nutritional status. I think this chapter has shown clearly why it is important, and therefore our goal should be to not forget the role of nutrition in our daily practice.

Suggested Reading

Arends J, Zuercher G, Dossett A, *et al*. Working group for developing the guidelines for parenteral nutrition of The German Association for Nutritional Medicine. Non-surgical oncology—Guidelines on parenteral nutrition. *Clin Nutr* 2006;**25**:245–59.

Clayson DB. Nutrition and experimental carcinogenesis: A review. *Cancer Res* 1997;**35**: 3292–300.

Galanti RM, Hansson L, Bergstrom R, *et al*. Diet and the risk of papillary and follicular thyroid carcinoma: A population-based case–control study in Sweden and Norway. *Cancer Causes Control* 1997:**8**:205–14.

Katergari SA, Milousis A, Pagonopoulou O, *et al*. Ghrelin in pathological conditions. *Endocr J* 2008;**55**:439–53.

Sciaudone MP, Chattopadhyay S, Freake HC. Chelation of zinc amplifies induction of growth hormone mRNA levels in cultured rat pituitary tumor cells. *J Nutr* 2000;**130**:158–63.

Szybinski Z, Jarosz M, Hubalewska-Dydejczyk A, *et al*. Iodine-deficiency prophylaxis and the restriction of salt consumption—a 21st century challenge. *Pol J Endocrinol* 2010;**1**:135–40.

Tulop OL, Krupp PP, Danforth E, *et al*. Characteristics of thyroid function in experimental protein malnutrition. *J Nutr* 1979;**109**:1321–32.

Wang H, Yang Z, Zhou B, *et al*. Fluoride-induced thyroid dysfunction in rats: Roles of dietary protein and calcium level. *Toxicol Ind Health* 2009;**25**:49–57.

Weimann A, Braga M, Harsanyi L, Laviano A, Ljungqvist O, Soeters P, DGEM (German Society for Nutritional Medicine), Jauch KW, Kemen M, Hiesmayr JM, Horbach T, Kuse ER, Vestweber KH, ESPEN (European Society for Parenteral and Enteral Nutrition): ESPEN guidelines on enteral nutrition: Surgery including organ transplantation. *Clin Nutr* 2006;**25**:224–44.

Patient Safety in Surgery for Thyroid Cancer

Amit Vats

This chapter describes the problem of human errors during surgical treatment of patients with thyroid cancer.

Introduction

In the United Kingdom, nine million surgical procedures were performed in 2008, of which >14,000 were surgeries on the thyroid and parathyroid glands. The exponential growth in the number of surgeries being performed in the past decades is due to improved surgical techniques, adjuvant therapies and better peri-operative care. Consequently, surgeries are being performed increasingly on extreme age groups with complex co-morbidities.

However, the rapid advances in surgical techniques are not matched by the quality, reliability and consistency of patient care. Studies have shown that ~10 % of patients admitted to acute-care hospitals suffer adverse events, of which surgery accounts for 40–50 %. Analysis of these adverse events reveals that nearly half of them are preventable.

Systems' View of Surgical Adverse Events

The WHO describes an adverse event as, 'An injury related to medical management, in contrast to complications of disease. Medical management includes all aspects of care, including diagnosis and treatment, failure to diagnose or treat, and the systems and equipment used to deliver care'.

A. Vats
Department of Biosurgery and Surgical Technology, Imperial College,
St Mary's Hospital, London, UK
e-mail: amit.vats@imperial.ac.uk

© The Author(s) 2012
F.L. Greene, A.L. Komorowski (eds.), *Clinical Approach to Well-differentiated Thyroid Cancers*, Head and Neck Cancer Clinics,
DOI 10.1007/978-81-322-2568-3_11

Traditionally, a surgeon's level of competence and the patient's comorbidities have been understood to be the cause of adverse patient outcomes. However, deeper examination of these adverse events reveals that many factors within a highly complex system are contributory. The complex interplay of organizational, cultural and team factors that constantly threaten safety lie hidden because of inherent defences in the system. However, albeit rarely, these hazards may go undetected and the lacunae in the system accumulate.

Surgical Adverse Events

Adverse events are common in surgery and can occur in any phase of the surgical care pathway. Thyroid and parathyroid surgery has been associated with an adverse event rate of 2.9 %. Some surgical adverse events are discussed below.

Wrong-Site Surgery

Wrong-site, wrong-procedure and wrong-person surgery is one such catastrophic event that should actually be considered to be a 'never' event. As the name suggests, these adverse events are 100 % preventable and hence should never occur. However rare such adverse events are, they have disastrous consequences for the patient, the surgical team and the hospital. Their incidence is difficult to estimate but it is likely that ~2500 cases of the 75 million surgical procedures performed per year in the USA constitute 'never' events. These reported incidents are merely the tip of the iceberg; many incidents are never reported.

Surgical Site Infection

Another preventable adverse event is surgical site infection (SSI). The SSI incidence after thyroid and parathyroid surgery is estimated to be between 0.25 and 2 %. Hospital guidelines give recommendations on the class and dose of prophylactic antibiotics that should be administered, and specify that, for maximal effectiveness, their administration should start within 60 min of the skin incision. However, this fact is often ignored. Studies have shown that compliance with guidelines for preventing SSI is as low as 50 %.

Thromboembolism

Deep vein thrombosis (DVT) and pulmonary embolism constitute 9 % of all adverse events. However, of note is the fact that they account for 19 % of negligent adverse events. Although guidelines for DVT prophylaxis are widely available, adherence to these guidelines can be as low as 30 %.

Causes of Adverse Events

Adverse events are a major concern to healthcare organizations and the reason for a number of malpractice lawsuits. Studies show that the vast majority of these events do not appear to be solely because of individual failure. Organizational factors, such as training, staffing, equipment support and failures in planning underlie these events. The poor interaction between team members and the lack of communication between various healthcare staff involved in patient care are other critical factors that are little recognized. Teamwork and communication between team members has largely been ignored as a fundamental aspect of surgical safety. Studies on communication in the operating theatre show absence of protocols and variation in their effectiveness. Failure of preoperative communication between surgeons and anaesthetists can lead to misidentification of patients and wrong-site surgery. The Joint Commission on Accreditation of Healthcare Organizations (JCAHO) found that 70 % of wrong-site surgeries are preventable by better communication between staff members.

In the absence of preoperative checks, crucial equipment and prostheses are often missing in most operating theatres. Equipment problems are more likely to cause distraction, disrupt workflow, delay case progression and lead to cancellations. Lack of communication between surgeons, nurses and anaesthetists can lead to omission of checks for ensuring patient safety. For example, the availability of blood and investigations, such as thyroid function tests, may not be checked prior to surgery, which could lead to complications during the intraoperative and postoperative periods. Unavailability of desired equipment is common in operating theatres and poor communication between surgeons and nurses is one of the prime reasons for these problems. Therefore, surgeons often have to adjust their technique and adapt the procedure to 'work around' the equipment problems, leading to technical errors. Attempts to follow guidelines, such as those for antibiotic and DVT prophylaxis, are impeded by blurred interprofessional responsibilities and ineffective communication. Therefore, guidelines or other similar interventions that fail to account for the wider system are unlikely to improve safety significantly. Once the surgery has been performed, the handover of information from the theatre team to ward staff can often be insufficient to ensure good patient care. This may lead to an omission of tasks, such as timely administration of antibiotics, blood investigations, removal of drains, etc.

How Do We Improve Patient Safety in Surgery?

Surgery is a complex system. Systems' problems need systems' solutions. Having a surgeon who is competent to perform a surgical procedure is important but not enough to ensure patient safety during surgery. To ensure good patient care, it is important that all the necessary information is communicated to appropriate staff members at the right time. Healthcare organizations and surgical teams are gradually coming to appreciate the importance of teamwork and communication in preventing surgical adverse events. In an attempt to prevent the occurrence of wrong-site events, JCAHO recommended the use of the 'universal' protocol, which is a three-step process consisting of patient verification, site marking and a preoperative 'time-out' to confirm the correct patient, side, site and procedure. It is mandatory in all organizations in the USA to perform a time-out prior to every surgical procedure. Over the past few months, a number of surgical teams and organizations have used this opportunity to develop an 'extended time-out' that incorporates a checklist with a pre-procedure team briefing. Recently, WHO has introduced a surgical safety checklist that ensures the carrying out of certain checks crucial to patient safety in operating theatres.

The Surgical Checklist

Checklists address human failures associated with omission. Omissions are most likely to occur with information overload and multiple steps in a process, and planned departures from routine processes. Checklists are used routinely in high reliability organizations, such as the aviation and nuclear power industries. In aviation, their use is mandatory for every stage of the flight. Pre-procedural briefings are also considered critical in other high reliability organizations as ways to improve safety by helping team members develop shared mental models of work and for the exchange of critical information. The items on surgical checklists currently in use in health organizations across the world generally consist of preoperative checks, some of which are confirmation of the site, side and surgery, availability of equipment, and the need for special investigations, etc. The teams also exchange patient- and procedure-related information and discuss any potential intraoperative events.

In January 2007, the World Alliance for Patient Safety began its work on the Second Global Patient Safety Challenge. They launched the 'Safe Surgery Saves Lives' project aimed at improving patient safety in surgery on a global scale. This international effort has resulted in the development of a WHO surgical checklist (Fig. 11.1, also available at http://www.who.int/patientsafety/safesurgery/tools_resources/SSSL_Checklist_finalJun08.pdf) that includes items to ensure the basic minimum of surgical safety checks; its application is intended to be global.

Improving team communication is another platform for ensuring all necessary checks by getting team members to discuss the surgical procedure and equipment needs, confirm patient identity and exchange information that may be relevant to postoperative patient care. The WHO checklist has been piloted at eight international sites across the eight WHO territories and has shown an improvement in patient safety processes, such as correct identification of the patient and timely use of prophylactic antibiotics. The use of checklists has also been shown to significantly reduce surgery-related morbidity and mortality.

SURGICAL SAFETY CHECKLIST (FIRST EDITION)

World Health Organization

Before induction of anaesthesia ▸▸▸▸▸▸▸▸▸   Before skin incision ▸▸▸▸▸▸▸▸▸▸▸   Before patient leaves operating room

SIGN IN

☐ PATIENT HAS CONFIRMED
  • IDENTITY
  • SITE
  • PROCEDURE
  • CONSENT

☐ SITE MARKED/NOT APPLICABLE

☐ ANAESTHESIA SAFETY CHECK COMPLETED

☐ PULSE OXIMETER ON PATIENT AND FUNCTIONING

DOES PATIENT HAVE A:

KNOWN ALLERGY?
☐ NO
☐ YES

DIFFICULT AIRWAY/ASPIRATION RISK?
☐ NO
☐ YES, AND EQUIPMENT/ASSISTANCE AVAILABLE

RISK OF >500ML BLOOD LOSS
(7ML/KG IN CHILDREN)?
☐ NO
☐ YES, AND ADEQUATE INTRAVENOUS ACCESS
  AND FLUIDS PLANNED

TIME OUT

☐ CONFIRM ALL TEAM MEMBERS HAVE
  INTRODUCED THEMSELVES BY NAME AND
  ROLE

☐ SURGEON, ANAESTHESIA PROFESSIONAL
  AND NURSE VERBALLY CONFIRM
  • PATIENT
  • SITE
  • PROCEDURE

ANTICIPATED CRITICAL EVENTS

☐ SURGEON REVIEWS: WHAT ARE THE
  CRITICAL OR UNEXPECTED STEPS,
  OPERATIVE DURATION, ANTICIPATED
  BLOOD LOSS?

☐ ANAESTHESIA TEAM REVIEWS: : ARE THERE
  ANY PATIENT-SPECIFIC CONCERNS?

☐ NURSING TEAM REVIEWS: HAS STERILITY
  (INCLUDING INDICATOR RESULTS) BEEN
  CONFIRMED? ARE THERE EQUIPMENT
  ISSUES OR ANY CONCERNS?

HAS ANTIBIOTIC PROPHYLAXIS BEEN GIVEN
WITHIN THE LAST 60 MINUTES?
☐ YES
☐ NOT APPLICABLE

IS ESSENTIAL IMAGING DISPLAYED?
☐ YES
☐ NOT APPLICABLE

SIGN OUT

☐ NURSE VERBALLY CONFIRMS WITH THE
  TEAM:

☐ THE NAME OF THE PROCEDURE RECORDED

☐ THAT INSTRUMENT, SPONGE AND NEEDLE
  COUNTS ARE CORRECT   (OR NOT
  APPLICABLE)

☐ HOW THE SPECIMEN IS LABELLED
  (INCLUDING PATIENT NAME)

☐ WHETHER THERE ARE ANY EQUIPMENT
  PROBLEMS TO BE ADDRESSED

☐ SURGEON, ANAESTHESIA PROFESSIONAL
  AND NURSE REVIEW THE KEY CONCERNS
  FOR RECOVERY AND MANAGEMENT
  OF THIS PATIENT

THIS CHECKLIST IS NOT INTENDED TO BE COMPREHENSIVE. ADDITIONS AND MODIFICATIONS TO FIT LOCAL PRACTICE ARE ENCOURAGED

Fig. 11.1 WHO surgical safety checklist

Operating Theatre Team Briefing

To facilitate team communication, develop a common understanding of the procedure and tasks between team members, and improve safety, pre-procedural briefings are considered critical in other high reliability organizations. Briefings in operating theatres are conducted before the start of the operating list. In the team briefing, the surgeons, nurses and anaesthetists discuss collectively the order of the patients on the list, the equipment required for the surgeries, and any anticipated problems or concerns. They can also discuss staffing and equipment problems. Briefings facilitate the transfer of critical information between people and create an atmosphere of openness, wherein team members feel empowered to contribute to the process. There is also some evidence that preoperative briefings contribute to an improvement in the safety culture and team environment within the operating theatre. Furthermore, preoperative briefings have been found to result in a reduction of equipment problems and an increase in staff morale.

Conclusion

In the operating theatre, checklists and briefings herald a change in the way we practise surgery. They would go a long way in improving teamwork, communication and, most importantly, patient safety. They help operating theatre teams to ensure that patient care is no longer susceptible to omissions, cultural and hierarchical barriers, and lapses in concentration in the busy and stressful environment. But this endeavour to develop a system that is consistent and reliable in providing care to patients depends upon the willingness of the surgeons and their teams to appreciate the importance of factors such as communication and teamwork, and adopt ways to mitigate adverse events that are secondary to systems failures.

Commentary

Andrzej L. Komorowski

Patient safety is clearly the cornerstone of every surgical procedure. The vast numbers of serious surgical adverse events are caused by simple, human errors, which can result in disastrous consequences. Yet, the risk of serious, even unthinkable, events can be lessened by some relatively simple actions, e.g. by repeatedly going over the checklists before every single procedure. This practice should be mandatory.

A key point made by the author is the problem of communication between team members. The ideal scenario would be for all team members to get along well, with the single aim of ensuring patient safety and welfare. Unfortunately, in the real world, surgeons have little say, if any, when it comes to staffing. It is also not uncommon to find that persons responsible for hospital staffing do not understand the specificity of the surgical entourage. To overcome these problems, surgeons would do well to follow Dr Vats' advice by using surgical checklists, time-outs and team debriefings, which would help teams to coordinate and minimize the risks of human error.

Finally, it is my personal opinion that prophylactic antibiotics are of little use in thyroid surgery. However, should antibiotic prophylaxis be initiated, it should be underlined that treatment should start 60 min before anaesthesia and not continued after the operation.

Suggested Reading

Gawande AA, Thomas EJ, Zinner MJ, *et al*. The incidence and nature of surgical adverse events in Colorado and Utah in 1992. *Surgery* 1999;**126**:66–75.

Haynes AB, Weiser TG, Berry WR, *et al*. A surgical safety checklist to reduce morbidity and mortality in a global population. *N Engl J Med* 2009;**360**:491–9.

Reason J. Human error: Models and management. *BMJ* 2000;**320**:768–70.

Vats A, Vincent CA, Nagpal K, *et al*. Practical challenges of introducing WHO surgical checklist: UK pilot experience. *BMJ* 2010;**340**:b5433.

Vincent C, Neale G, Woloshynowych M. Adverse events in British hospitals: Preliminary retrospective record review. *BMJ* 2001;**322**:517–19.

Pietro Iacconi and Carmine De Bartolomeis

All complications that may occur during or after surgical treatment of thyroid cancer are summarized in this chapter. Prophylactic measures that lower the risks of these complications and the management of the immediate postoperative as well as long-term complications are discussed.

Introduction

Thyroid surgery has progressed significantly since the nineteenth century when half or more of the patients undergoing this operation died from it. Currently, thyroidectomy is a very safe operation which has an associated mortality rate approaching zero. The morbidity associated with thyroid surgery is also very low. Nevertheless, the complications of thyroidectomy remain a matter of concern, especially as thyroid disease often occurs in young patients whose life expectancy is expected to be long. Most complications associated with thyroidectomy can be minimized or even avoided by an experienced thyroid surgeon. The surgeon is an important prognostic factor with his 'manner' or 'style' of technical performance. In-depth knowledge of the anatomy of the central neck compartment and meticulous surgical technique are essential to protect the vital structures of the neck.

General Complications

As with most operations, the complications associated with thyroidectomy can be listed as general and local. General complications include cardiac and pulmonary problems, gastrointestinal dysfunction such as nausea, vomiting and ileus, and renal

P. Iacconi (✉) • C. De Bartolomeis
Department of Surgery, University of Pisa, Ospedale Santa Chiara, Pisa, Italy
e-mail: p.iacconi@med.unipi.it

© The Author(s) 2012
F.L. Greene, A.L. Komorowski (eds.), *Clinical Approach to Well-differentiated Thyroid Cancers*, Head and Neck Cancer Clinics,
DOI 10.1007/978-81-322-2568-3_12

and urinary tract problems. The general problems that occur with thyroidectomy are related to the underlying thyroid disease, the patient's associated medical conditions, and to the general anaesthetic rather than to the procedure itself. These non-surgery related problems are all relatively rare and occur in 1–2 % of patients in large reported series of thyroidectomies. Arrhythmias are the most common cardiac complications and occur in patients with hyperthyroidism or with an underlying cardiac disease. Pulmonary problems are infrequent, considering the extensive manipulation of the upper airway during thyroidectomy. Atelectasia, bronchitis or pneumonia occur in <1 % of patients. Respiratory compromise can also occur with tracheal collapse from chondromalacia or kinking of a soft, tortuous trachea. These problems are rare and usually occur with long-standing large multinodular goitres that have compressed the trachea and have recurred frequently after previous operations. When the thyroid is removed, the trachea can collapse or kink because of loss of integrity of the cartilagineous rings. In this situation, the thyroid gland was acting as an external support for the trachea even though the gland had compressed and compromised the cartilaginous integrity of the rings. Tracheostomy is the standard treatment if a soft trachea is encountered after prolonged endotracheal intubation. External splinting of the trachea with Marlex™ mesh (Davol, Inc. Warwick, RI, USA) has also been used in this setting. Some surgeons use splinting of the trachea with two stitches (one for each side), which are ligated onto a dental roll on the skin.

Postoperative nausea with or without vomiting can occur in as many as 10–15 % of patients. This troublesome problem is anaesthesia-related and can be substantially lessened by effective antiemetic prophylaxis.

Specific Complications

The major specific complications of thyroidectomy include postoperative cervical haemorrhage, airway obstruction, recurrent laryngeal nerve (RLN) injury and hypoparathyroidism. Thyroid crisis in patients with hyperthyroidism who are inadequately prepared for surgery is a serious complication, which nowadays is of historic importance.

Haemorrhage

Samuel Gross, a leading American surgeon of the late nineteenth century, described thyroid surgery as 'butchery' because of the high mortality related to uncontrolled bleeding and haemorrhagic complications. Despite ongoing refinements in techniques, innovations in surgical instruments and a better understanding of underlying thyroid disorders, postoperative haematoma remains, fortunately, an uncommon but potentially serious complication of thyroid surgery.

Post-thyroidectomy haemorrhage has an incidence that varies in the literature from 0.49 to 4.3 %. Clots compressing the rigid cartilaginous trachea can compromise airflow in a few cases. Moreover, impairment in venous and lymphatic drainage with resultant laryngopharyngeal oedema may place the patient's airway at significant risk. The patient may present with respiratory distress, pain or pressure sensation in the neck, or dysphagia. Signs include progressive neck swelling, dyspnoea and/or stridor and, possibly, significant drain tube losses. The aetiology of haematoma formation includes slipping of ligatures, re-opening of previously cauterized veins, or bleeding from residual thyroid parenchyma. The time frame within which it may occur also varies, but the majority of haemorrhagic symptoms occur early in the postoperative period, i.e. within 6 h of the intervention.

Risk factors associated with postoperative haemorrhage are related to the patient, to the underlying thyroid pathology and to the surgeon. The first group includes patients with haemophilia, von Willebrand disease and chronic renal failure; iatrogenic bleeding results from the use of anticoagulant medications, such as those that inhibit vitamin K-dependent coagulation factors or act against platelet function. Similarly, smokers have a recognized increase in bleeding tendency. Particular risks associated with the underlying thyroid pathology have been postulated. The increased vascularity of the thyroid in patients with Basedow disease and toxic multinodular glands has been well documented. The efficacy of Lugol iodine in decreasing blood flow of the thyroid parenchyma in these conditions has been proven. Intrathoracic goitres and reoperations also have a greater propensity for postoperative bleeding.

Surgical technique plays a strong role in preventing postoperative bleeding. Sections of the strap muscles may be a source of potential bleeding unless they are adequately ligated or coagulated. Care should also be taken when elevating subplatysmal flaps or closing vertically divided strap muscles to avoid injury to the anterior jugular veins. Anaesthetic technique is also important in haematoma prevention. A smooth extubation without significant coughing or retching, and controlling both postoperative vomiting and pain avoids a rise in venous and arterial pressures which, in turn, minimize the risk of postoperative bleeding. Positioning of the patient in a head-up position lowers venous pressures throughout the course of the procedure. Several manoeuvres have been advocated to assist in the recognition of potential bleeding points by raising the venous pressure prior to closure of the neck wound:

• Putting the patient in the Trendelenburg position (head-down tilt)
• Pushing on the epigastrium of the patient (similar to the Valsalva manoeuvre)

Recent reports in the international literature suggest that drains should not be used as a preventive measure; however, if used, they may signal evidence of bleeding.

Numerous technical advances have taken place since Kocher's refinement of thyroidectomy. Diathermy with the use of monopolar or bipolar electrosurgery provides useful haemostasis for small vessels that previously would have been tied manually. Vessel ligating clips have also proved an alternative to traditional ligatures. Their holding strength has been studied and proven mainly in animal models (and in renal vessels in humans). However, the clips can nevertheless potentially dislodge, which results in bleeding. More recent alternative measures, such as the Ligasure™ (Covidien AG, Valleylab, Boulder CO, USA) and Harmonic Scalpel™ (Ethicon Endo-Surgery

Inc, Blue Ash OH, USA), have been used increasingly for thyroid surgery. At present, it appears that both instruments significantly reduce operating time while remaining as safe for standard vessel ligation. In the case of Ligasure™, one study has demonstrated that the vessel sealed with this device can withstand three times the normal systolic blood pressure. Unlike conventional diathermy, this seal does not rely on a proximal thrombus and eschar formation, both of which may become dislodged under certain conditions. In other fields of surgery, they have been shown to reduce operative blood loss and postoperative complications. The use of oxidized cellulose, e.g. Surgicel™ (Johnson and Johnson, New Brunswick, NJ, USA) or other bioabsorbable topical haemostatic agents, may be useful and facilitate haemostasis, both by mechanical tissue pressure when inserted, similar to a sponge, or by promoting blood cells and larger particles to form a coagulum within the interstices of the cellulose, converting it into an impermeable, relatively heavy patch.

Only a small group of patients with minimal swelling, lack of symptoms and no progression of haematoma should be considered for conservative management. However, an expeditious re-intervention is advocated strongly upon suspicion of haematoma formation, given the potentially life-threatening sequelae of this complication. Tachycardia, sweating, irritability and confusion are early signs of hypoxia that imply a full alert for neck swelling, drainage and obvious signs of airway obstruction to avoid delays in re-intervention. It is important to ensure a surgical presence within the operating theatre during the extubation and recovery period. Evidence of bleeding in this period requires an immediate return to the theatre. Evidence of progressive bleeding within the first few hours after surgery should also mandate a re-exploration. In the event of significant airway compromise developing rapidly and in the absence of staff appropriately trained in intubation, bedside evacuation of the haematoma may be necessary. It is insufficient to remove the superficial skin sutures and those closing the platysma alone; it is mandatory to open the linea alba to decompress the neck. It should always be kept in mind that an inability to secure an adequate airway via intubation may result in the need for a surgical airway to be established via a tracheostomy. Similarly, persistent laryngeal oedema post-evacuation may necessitate prolonged intubation and treatment with systemic steroids. At the time of surgical re-intervention, attention to the parathyroids and the RLN should be paid because these structures are vulnerable to injury or removal during the process of irrigation, suction and clot evacuation. Blind clamping of vessels within the haematoma has to be avoided. It is a well-recognized phenomenon that sometimes no discrete point of bleeding can be identified; should this be the case, closure should ensue after ensuring that all potential sources have been adequately explored. Our group routinely leaves two suction drains at the end of exploration.

Nerve Injury

Paralysis of the RLN is the most common complication after a thyroid operation. The nerves supplying the larynx and the pharyngeal constrictors arise from the nucleus ambiguous and course through the vagus nerve. The RLNs and the superior laryngeal nerves are branches of the ipsilateral vagus nerves. Each RLN supplies all of the intrinsic ipsilateral muscles of the larynx, the cricopharyngeal muscles, and sensation to the laryngeal mucosa below the vocal cords. The superior laryngeal nerve has two branches: the internal laryngeal nerve, which supplies ipsilateral sensation above the true vocal cords, and external laryngeal nerve, which gives motor supply to the ipsilateral external cricothyroid muscles. The RLN usually tracks upward in the neck in the tracheo-oesophageal groove medial to the carotid artery. Its course is often more oblique on the right and more vertical on the left. The recurrent nerves cross the lower lateral border of the thyroid at the level at which the inferior thyroid artery enters the gland. Most commonly, they pass behind the artery but can also course anterior to it. The nerves then course behind the lobe and through or behind the Berry ligament before penetrating the cricothyroid muscle to enter the larynx. The location and course of the RLN can show a great deal of individual anatomical variation. In ~1 % of the population, the right RLN is non-recurrent and enters the larynx from a superior or lateral position. Likewise, it is not always a single strand and its pattern of branching can be variable. The normal location of the RLNs and their common anatomical variations must be understood and kept in mind when performing thyroidectomy.

Complications involving the RLNs cause considerable morbidity. Although injury to a single nerve can remain asymptomatic, patients are more likely to have temporary or permanent hoarseness. RLN injury associated with thyroidectomy has decreased progressively. Although it should occur in <1 % of patients who undergo thyroidectomy, it probably still occurs in 5 % of patients. The rate of RLN injury during reoperations is significantly higher compared with that after initial operations, with an incidence ranging from 1 % to as high as 24 %. The main reason for the improved results is that the current recommended surgical approach identifies the nerve and protects it throughout the course of the dissection. If the RLN has been stretched or roughly handled, neurapraxia may occur, which can last for up to 6 months while the nerve regenerates along the intact axon sheath. If the nerve is transected inadvertently, permanent hoarsness will occur. If this complication is recognized intraoperatively the nerve should be re-anastomosed using microsurgical techniques. If, in order to allow a tension-free anastomosis, too large a segment of a nerve is missing, a nerve graft can be used. The ansa cervicalis is generally the most frequently used donor nerve. The ansa's branch to the lower portion of the sternothyroid muscle is identified and dissected toward its muscular termination inferiorly A nerve stimulator can be used to help identify the ansa, but is usually not required. A sufficient length of the nerve is harvested to allow for a tension-free anastomosis between the ends of the nerve graft and the RLN. The microneural anastomosis is performed with 10-0 nylon sutures with the aid of an operation microscope.

If the patient is hoarse in the postoperative period, it is likely that this will be temporary if the nerve was identified and noted to be intact during the operation. The chance of recovery is high and the patient should be observed for at least 6 months for spontaneous recovery to occur. With isolated unilateral injury, if the position of the paralysed vocal cord is midline and compensation by the contralateral cord is effective, the damage may not be recognized until some point later, when weakness or change in the voice becomes apparent. After a 6–12-month period, the injury is considered to be permanent and a number of measures can help lessen hoarseness. These include speech therapy, teflon injection into the vocal cord, nerve anastomoses and other more sophisticated surgical procedures.

If bilateral RLN injury occurs, the main effect is often on the competency of the airway, and the voice may remain surprisingly close to normal. If bilateral nerve injury manifests as stridor on extubation, the diagnosis is obvious and the patient must be treated with reintubation or tracheostomy. However, the manifestation can be delayed if the vocal cords are in a persistently abducted position after operation because of the splinting effect of the endotracheal tube. These patients can then be diagnosed later with dyspnoea and stridor.

A vocal cord lateralization procedure can be performed if the injury has been present for >1 year. A teflon paste or silicon can be injected into the flaccid vocal cord. Vocal cord injection improves both the volume and the tone of speech. The material is injected in the vocal corn process anterior and lateral to the margin of the fold. Sufficient material is injected to swell the cord to the midline and restore phonation. A thyroplasty that medializes the paralysed cord can be performed. The indications for a thyroplasty are unilateral or bilateral vocal cord paralysis or paresis, incomplete glottis closure, and vocal fold bowing. This procedure can be performed in various ways. Re-innervation techniques have been attempted, with variable results. Because re-innervation of the paralysed laryngeal muscles takes at least 3 months, vocal cord injection is recommended to improve the speech during the interim period. With bilateral nerve injury, the main concern is to provide an adequate airway. Generally, a tracheostomy is required in this situation. Recovery of nerve function can take as long as 6–12 months. In the absence of an improvement after this period, a permanent tracheostomy tube with a speaking valve is an option. Otherwise, the vocal fold can be moved laterally to restore an adequate airway. This alters the voice and results in abnormal speech. A compromise must be made between a reasonably acceptable voice and a patent airway.

Intraoperative RLN monitoring can help the surgeon in protecting the recurrent nerve (*see* Chap. 7). Even if a variety of intraoperative RLN monitoring methods are available, they are all based on the visual or acoustic registration of evoked electromyography of the laryngeal muscles. Primarily, the registered activity proves conductivity of the stimulated nerve segment towards the muscle, so that stimulation distal to the lesion should show persistent electromyographic response. This technology is usually not used in our department. The superior laryngeal nerve can be injured when taking down the superior pole of the ipsilateral thyroid lobe. This nerve is not always visible during open classical thyroidectomy, whereas it is often easily visible during minimally invasive thyroidectomy through the magnifying lens. Its injury will lead to subtle loss of voice pitch and voice volume. The patient will complain of voice weakness and voice change. This is a serious matter for professional singers, as was shown by the classical and controversial clinical case of a famous soprano who was unable to sing after a thyroid operation at the beginning of the nineteenth century. When bilateral injury occurs, patients can experience swallowing disorders and be susceptible to aspiration.

The superior laryngeal nerves are damaged in 0.3–2 % of patients who undergo thyroidectomy. This is likely to be a low estimate, as the complication is probably underreported because of the subtlety of its symptoms.

Rarely, the cervical sympathetic trunk may be damaged during thyroidectomy. This will result in Horner syndrome. This is an unusual complication but can occur with very large glands, invasive tumours, or with reoperations when scar tissue has obliterated the normal tissue planes. Injury to the spinal accessory nerve can occur with neck dissections when combined with thyroidectomy, but should not occur with thyroidectomy alone.

Other local injures to the oesophagus, trachea, thoracic duct, jugular vein, carotid artery and spinal accessory nerve are also rare and usually occur when dealing with invasive tumours, reoperations and performing associated neck dissection.

Hypocalcaemia

The incidence of parathyroid gland injury is related to the extent of the thyroidectomy and to the experience of the surgeon. The incidence of permanent hypoparathyroidism after total thyroidectomy ranges from 0.7 to 2 % but some authors suggest that transient, asymptomatic hypocalcaemia occurs in most patients undergoing thyroidectomy. This statement is true in settings such as a reoperation, in which the risks of injury to these structures are greater from scarring and distorted anatomy. Postoperative hypoparathyroidism may result from the inadvertent removal of the parathyroid glands along with the thyroid. More commonly, it is caused by devascularization of the parathyroid glands during ligation of the blood supply to the thyroid gland. It is essential to ligate the branches of the inferior thyroid artery close to the thyroid capsule to preserve the vascular supply to each parathyroid gland, as the parathyroid glands in most people derive their blood supply from this artery. These vessels are delicate and can be injured by blind suctioning in the operative field or by careless efforts to control bleeding by imprecise clamping or suturing the tissues. The operative field should be kept dry by blotting with wet, sterile gauze so that the parathyroids can be identified and their vascular supply preserved. Symptoms of acute postoperative hypocalcaemia usually develop within the first 24 h. Numbness and tingling starts around the mouth and then progresses to the hands, fingers, feet and toes.

A positive Chvostek sign (twitching of the ipsilateral lip when tapping over the facial nerve) and a positive Trousseau sign (development of carpal spasm when a blood pressure cuff is placed around the arm with the pressure between systolic and diastolic values for 5 min) are often present. If untreated, carpal pedal spasm, tetany and life-threatening cardiac arrhythmias may occur; symptom occurrence is variable and depends on the rate and decrement of the drop in ionized calcium. The incidence of hypoparathyroidism can be diminished substantially by the use of parathyroid autotransplantation. There is no reason to hope that a damaged parathyroid gland will recover its function. Autotransplantation is a much more reliable technique when aiming at preserving the parathyroid's viability. The capsule of ischaemic glands should be incised to see whether they change colour. If they remain dark, they are transplanted in a muscle pocket in the ipsilateral sternocleido-mastoid muscle. After the operation, serum calcium, magnesium and phosphorus levels should be measured. The diagnosis of hypocalcaemia should be based on ionized calcium levels if there is any question about the patient's circulating total protein and albumin status. If the total serum calcium is <8 mg/dl, vitamin D replacement therapy should be initiated with 1α-hydroxyl cholecalciferol. Mild postoperative hypocalcaemia can generally be treated with oral calcium supplementation. Symptomatic hypocalcaemia requires more aggressive treatment, and intra-venous calcium may be necessary. If hypocalcaemia is caused by the hungry bone syndrome, the serum phosphorus level will also be low. If hypocalcaemia and hyperphosphataemia remain after a year, permanent hypoparathyroidism is present and the patient will require long-term therapy with oral calcium and vitamin D. Permanent hypoparathyroidism is a serious, lifelong disability that requires regular monitoring of serum calcium levels and adjustments in replacement therapy. Fatigue, paraesthesias, irritability and cataract formation are common continuing problems. In thyroid surgery, the choice of a skilled endocrine surgeon using a meticulous technique to preserve well-vascularized parathyroid glands in the neck and liberal use of parathyroid autotransplantation will effectively limit the rate of permanent hypoparathyroidism with thyroid surgery including a total thyroidectomy (*see also* Chap. 7).

Other Specific Complications

Inadvertent tracheal perforation during traditional thyroid operations, in general, is rarely reported. Forgotten goitre is extremely rare; it is frequently an upper mediastinal thyroid mass found after total tyroidectomy It is most often the consequence of incomplete removal of a plunging goitre, but can also be caused by an aberrant thyroid in the mediastinum. I remember at least two of my patients operated for a 'total' thyroidectomy with a residue in the neck (one required reoperation), and one more with an aberrant thyroid in the mediastinum. Sometimes a forgotten goitre is because of a 'grapelike goitre', which can mislead the surgeon in finding the correct dissection plane.

The number of patients undergoing endoscopic thyroid surgery is increasing rapidly because of the excellent cosmetic results, early recovery and reduced tissue trauma. However, it is important to recognize that surgery for a benign thyroid nodule might lead to implantation of thyroid cells, and this complication is not uncommon with subcutaneous implantation of an adenomatous goitre. Thus, precaution against rupture of a nodule, such as avoiding cutting or morselization of the nodule, should be carefully considered during endoscopic surgery even in patients with a benign thyroid nodule. Cosmetic appearance is of major importance, especially as thyroidectomies often involve young women. Achieving an optimal cosmetic result is easiest when one applies a number of principles, including elements normally associated with plastic surgery, such as orientation of the skin incision. This need favoured the ascent of minimally invasive thyroid surgery. Unfortunately, the edges of the wound can be traumatized by the excessive traction used in the mini-invasive thyroid approach, in which one can be forced to resect the margins of the wound. Infection and seroma formation are extremely uncommon in such operations. Some fluid can be aspirated with a fine needle but it is often unnecessary (for more information on minimally invasive thyroid procedures, *see* Chap. 8).

Commentary

Andrzej M. Wysocki

The initial thyroid surgeries, performed >100 years ago, were loaded with serious risks of general and local complications, the most common being bleeding and infection. Although today these complications are rare, bleeding, hypoparathyroidism and laryngeal nerve injury are still a cause for concern.

The complication rate increases with increasing size of the thyroid mass and also with the extent of the operation. Complications (mostly hypoparathyroidism and laryngeal nerve injury) increase, after total thyroidectomy or thyroid lobectomy (especially with lymphadenectomy) than after a simple goitre resection.

A particularly dangerous complication is postoperative bleeding, which develops within the first few hours in a closed space and can result in a haematoma compressing the upper airways. The dominating symptom is dyspnoea. The blood coming out of drains may not be enough to prevent tracheal compression. The bleeding is not likely to cause hypotension either. In this life-threatening situation it is necessary to open a wound immediately, sometimes even at the bedside, and remove the haematoma. The bleeding vessel can later be identified in the operating theatre and precise haemostasis performed. It is not always possible to find a source of bleeding during this emergency operation. However, the bleeding may never return. Before the operation, the surgeon must bear in mind that many patients who take widely used anticoagulants and antiplatelet drugs continuously may not mention this to their doctor. A gentle tissue dissection and precise haemostasis are indispensible elements during each thyroidectomy. It is not possible to eliminate completely the risk of postoperative bleeding in this procedure. In my opinion, this is the reason why two suction drains should be left in the operation field after performing each thyroid surgery, even when the haemostasis is perfect. Also, a careful dissection reduces the rate of laryngeal nerve injury and hypoparathyroidism. It is possible to adhere to these simple rules when the operation field remains clear and visible. It is more difficult during reoperation, when scars and fibrosis cover the view or while searching for a bleeding vessel during reoperation. This situation is also complicated when it is difficult to have a good view of the operating field, for instance, in retrosternal goitre.

Extensive thyroidectomy, especially in the case of undifferentiated thyroid carcinoma, may cause even rare injuries such as cervical sympathetic chain damage causing Horner syndrome, or cervical oesophagus damage. Extensive thyroidectomy may also cause lymphorrhoea, which usually subsides in 3–4 weeks after introducing conservative therapy of total parenteral nutrition and octreotide instead of oral feeding. The thyroid's entire hormonal function ceases after total thyroidectomy. It is not a complication but a consequence of the extensiveness of the operation; the patient requires continuous hormonal treatment.

The surgeon's experience in mitigating the general complications of thyroid surgery cannot be overemphasized. The most effective way to reduce the complication rate is to train surgeons who initially should be accompanied by an expert until he or she gains the necessary experience to be self-reliant. This is not to say that complications will not occur with the most experienced surgeons, but they can certainly be lessened.

Suggested Reading

Bellantone R, Lombardi CP, Raffaelli M, et al. Is routine supplementation therapy (calcium and vitamin D) useful after total thyroidectomy? Surgery 2002;**132:**1109–13.

Burkey SH, van Heerden JA, Thompson GB, et al. Re-exploration for symptomatic hematomas after cervical exploration. Surgery 2001;**130:**914–20.

Defechereux T, Hamoir E, Nguyen Dang D, et al. Le drainage en chirurgie thyroïdienne: est-ce toujours une necessité ? Ann Chir 1997;**51:**647–52.

Gosnell JE, Campbell P, Sidhu S, et al. Inadvertent tracheal perforation during thyroidectomy. Br J Surg 2006;**93:**55–6.

Lenquist S, Cahlin C, Smeds S. The superior laryngeal nerve in thyroid surgery. Surgery 1987;**102:**999–1008.

Reeve T, Thompson NW. Complications of thyroid surgery: How to avoid them, how to manage them, and observation on their possible effect on the whole patient. World J Surg 2000;**24:**971–5.

Randolph GW. Surgical anatomy of the recurrent laryngeal nerve. In: Randolph GW (ed.). Surgery of the thyroid and parathyroid glands. Philadelphia, PA: Saunders; 2003:300–42.

Randolph G, Kobler J, Wilkins J. Recurrent laryngeal nerve identification and assessment during thyroid surgery: Laryngeal palpation. World J Surg 2004;**28:**755–60.

Rosato L, Avenia N, Bernante P, et al. Complication of thyroid surgery: Analysis of a multicentric study on 14934 patients operated in Italy over 5 years. World J Surg 2004;**28:**271–6.

Terris DJ, Seybt MW, Elcchoufi M, et al. Cosmetic thyroid surgery: Defining the essential principles. Laryngoscope 2007;**117:**1168–72.

Barbara Jarząb and Daria Handkiewicz-Junak

This chapter first reviews briefly how to assess patient prognosis after completion of surgery and thereafter how to tailor medical treatment and follow up.

Introduction

Effective treatment and follow up of differentiated thyroid cancer (DTC) begins with an assessment of the risk of recurrence or death from the disease, depending on the individual characteristics of patients and their tumours. Once patient prognosis is established, treatment and follow up can be finely tailored. In a substantial number of patients, post-surgical treatment will include adjuvant radioiodine and some will need external beam irradiation. A small group of patients with advanced, disseminated disease and very poor prognosis will be good candidates for clinical trials due to lack of standard treatments. Lastly, all patients will require levothyroxine (L-T4) therapy, but the degree of thyroid-stimulating hormone (TSH) suppression will depend on the prognostic group the patient is assigned to.

Prognostic Factors in Differentiated Thyroid Cancer

Therapeutic strategies depend on factors that influence the prognosis. As in other cancers, numerous studies on DTC have concentrated on relatively simple clinico-pathological prognostic factors (Table 13.1), such as the patient's age at diagnosis, sex, primary tumour size, extent of disease, or pathological histotype, to formulate risk group stratification or staging systems.

B. Jarząb • D. Handkiewicz-Junak (✉)
Department of Nuclear Medicine and Endocrine Oncology, Maria Skłodowska-Curie
Memorial Cancer Center and Institute of Oncology, Gliwice Branch, Gliwice, Poland
e-mail: dhandkiewicz@io.gliwice.pl

© The Author(s) 2012
F.L. Greene, A.L. Komorowski (eds.), *Clinical Approach to Well-differentiated Thyroid Cancers*, Head and Neck Cancer Clinics,
DOI 10.1007/978-81-322-2568-3_13

Table 13.1 Clinical prognostic factors used in staging systems for differentiated thyroid cancer

Factor	Positive prognostic indicator	Negative prognostic indicator
Patient-related factors		
Age	Younger (usually <40/45 years of age)	Older
Gender	Female	Male
Tumour-related factors		
Histopathology	Poorly differentiated	Well differentiated
	PTC: Classical, follicular variant	PTC: Tall cell, columnar cell
	FTC: Minimally invasive	FTC: Widely invasive, poorly differentiated
Primary tumour—diameter	Small (the best prognosis for tumours of ≤1 cm)	Large
Primary tumour—extension beyond thyroid capsule	No	Yes
Lymph node metastasis	Absent	Present
Distant metastases	Absent	Present
Treatment-related factors		
Surgical resection	Total thyroidectomy and appropriate extent of lymphadenectomy	Incomplete removal of cancer tissues and/or lack of total thyroidectomy and of appropriate extent of lymphadenectomy

FTC follicular thyroid cancer, *PTC* papillary thyroid cancer

Age at diagnosis is an independent prognostic factor in DTC. According to the TNM (tumour, node, metastasis) staging (*see* Chap. 5), all patients ≤45 years of age who are diagnosed without distant metastases are considered to have stage I disease, i.e. they belong to the 'low-risk' group. Older patients suffer from more locally aggressive tumours, higher incidence of distant metastases and more aggressive histopathological variants of thyroid cancer. Also, the incidence of recurrences is higher and earlier after the initial treatment compared with that in younger patients. On the other hand, evidence shows that children <15 years of age have a pattern of tumour recurrence and distant metastases that is similar to that of adults (>60 years of age). Children commonly present with more advanced tumour stage than adults and have more cancer recurrences after therapy, but often live for many years after recurrence. Fortunately, an increasing body of evidence also shows that if properly treated, the recurrence rate in children can be low, and the high recurrence rate reported in the earlier studies can be attributed to suboptimal treatment in children with DTC. Two other patient-related factors—male gender and familial papillary thyroid cancer (PTC)—have been reported in some series.

Tumour burden, which takes into account not only size and extent of the primary tumour but also the presence and size of local or distant metastases, is a prognostic factor of utmost importance. Although both T and N status can be assessed preoperatively using neck ultrasound or computed tomography (CT), it is the histo-pathological examination of surgical specimens that provides doctors with the most accurate method of staging, known as pTNM (p = pathological). The importance of primary tumour size and its invasiveness has been proved in many studies. A direct relationship exists between the size of the primary tumour and the risk of recurrence and cancer-specific mortality. This relationship does not refer to papillary microcarcinoma. If the tumour is <1 cm, the prognosis is excellent both in terms of relapse-free and overall survival after surgery without any adjuvant treatment, except for L-T4 substitution. Approximately 5–10 % of tumours grow directly into the surrounding neck tissues, increasing both morbidity and mortality. Local invasion can range from microscopic invasion beyond the thyroid capsule to gross cancer infiltration of the surrounding tissues, involving the oesophagus and trachea. Microscopic invasion into the surrounding tissues has a much better prognosis than a macroscopic tumour invading contiguous structures (*see also* Chap. 9). Wide, especially if macroscopic, invasion is a poor prognostic factor both in PTC and follicular thyroid cancer (FTC), exposing patients to a higher recurrence rate, distant metastases and cancer-related mortality. Although not considered in TNM staging and in only a few other staging systems (e.g. European Organization for Research and Treatment of Cancer, EORTC), less differentiated cancers are associated with a poor prognosis. Also, some variants of PTC (e.g. solid or tall cell) and FTC (e.g. widely invasive) carry a worse prognosis. Molecular prognostic factors have not yet been widely accepted in DTC. However, cell ploidy which has been included in DNA ploidy Age, Metastases, Extent, Size (DAMES) staging, and *BRAF* mutation are now arousing increased interest as a negative prognostic factor.

Distant metastases, although diagnosed in <10 % of patients with DTC, carry an inevitably poor prognosis with a 5-year cancer-specific mortality of ~40 %. The outcome is influenced mainly by the patient's age, the tumour's metastatic site, ability to concentrate radioiodine (^{131}I) and tumour bulk. Survival is longest with diffuse microscopic lung metastases diagnosed only on post-treatment ^{131}I imaging and not by X-ray. So, although it is difficult to prove in clinical studies, the earlier ^{131}I treatment for metastatic disease is initiated, the better the chance for a good response. The prognosis is the worst when metastases do not concentrate ^{31}I or appear as large lung nodules. The prognostic importance of regional lymph node metastases is controversial, yet an increasingly number of studies find nodal metastases to be a risk factor for local tumour recurrence, distant metastasis and cancer-specific mortality, especially if there are bilateral cervical or mediastinal lymph node metastases, or if the tumour invades through the lymph node capsule.

In addition to patient- or tumour-related prognostic factors, a persistent or recurrent local thyroid cancer may be also due to inadequate initial surgery, because the surgical protocol was incomplete. Recurrence rates are high with large thyroid gland remnants. Some studies have found that patients treated by lobectomy alone have a 5–10 % recurrence rate in the opposite thyroid lobe and an overall long-term recurrence rate of >30 % (versus 1 % after total thyroidectomy and ^{131}I therapy). Total thyroidectomy was also shown to increase disease-free survival as an independent prognostic factor in multivariate analysis.

Table 13.2 Differentiated thyroid cancer risk stratification according to the American Thyroid Association guidelines and European Consensus

American Thyroid Association	European consensus
Low-risk patients	
No local or distant metastases and all macroscopic tumour resected and no tumour invasion of loco-regional tissues or structures; the tumour does not have aggressive histology (e.g. tall cell, insular, columnar cell carcinoma) or vascular invasion. If ^{131}I treatment is given, ^{131}I uptake does not occur outside the thyroid bed on the first post-treatment RxWBS[a]	Complete surgery and favourable histology, and unifocal tumour of >1 cm, N0, M0 and no extrathyroidal extension[a]
Intermediate-risk patients	
Microscopic invasion of tumour into perithyroidal soft tissues at initial surgery, or cervical lymph node metastases, or ^{131}I uptake outside the thyroid bed on the RxWBS done after thyroid remnant ablation, or tumour with aggressive histology or vascular invasion	<Total thyroidectomy, or no lymph node dissection, or age <18 years, or T1 > 1 cm and T2, N0 M0
High-risk patients	
Macroscopic tumour invasion, or incomplete tumour resection, or distant metastases, or possibly thyroglobulinaemia out of proportion to what is seen on the post-treatment scan	Distant metastases, or incomplete tumour resection, or complete tumour resection but high risk for recurrence or mortality; tumour extension beyond the thyroid capsule (T3 or T4), or lymph node involvement

RxWBS diagnostic whole-body scan
[a]All factors must be present

On the basis of combined analysis of prognostic factors, prognostic scoring systems were developed to stratify high- and low-risk DTC patients. At least 18 staging systems for PTC, FTC or both have been formulated on the basis of retrospective patient outcome evaluations. In all these studies, the primary endpoint was survival, and recurrence was not considered. This is the best approach in cancers with a high mortality rate. However, in DTC, in which almost 90 % of patients do not die of the cancer, recurrence-free survival should also be an important factor when considering the best approach to treatment. For assessment of the risk of recurrence, three-level stratification was developed by the American Thyroid Association. A similar stratification was used by the European Consensus to establish an indication for adjuvant radioiodine treatment in DTC. It is generally agreed that patients with tumours <1 cm, which are not locally invaded and which have a favourable histopathology (Table 13.2), constitute the low-risk category. On the other hand, patients with distant metastases, widely invasive local disease and elevated postoperative thyroglobulin (Tg) level constitute the other end of the disease spectrum, i.e. the high-risk group. It is also generally agreed that adjuvant treatment can be avoided in the first group whereas it is necessary in the latter group. However, the largest group constitutes patients in the 'grey zone' (the intermediate-risk group) for which the indication for postoperative adjuvant treatment is highly debatable.

Non-surgical Treatment of Differentiated Thyroid Cancer

Radioiodine Ablation of Thyroid Remnants

Radioiodine remains the mainstay of postoperative treatment and has been used for >60 years in DTC patients. It is applied both in patients without any signs of persistent disease as an adjunct to surgical treatment, and in patients with disseminated or locally inoperable disease. In the first case, radioiodine treatment has to ablate any residual normal thyroid tissue in order to facilitate follow up and early detection of persistent or recurrent disease by measurement of serum Tg (with or without TSH stimulation) or radioactive iodine scanning. Traditionally, this kind of radioiodine treatment has been called 'thyroid ablation'; this term will be used throughout this chapter. However, the goal of ablation is also to destroy any residual microscopical thyroid cancer in an effort to decrease the risk of recurrence and disease-specific mortality; in this setting, it is a typical adjuvant cancer treatment. Radioiodine is also used to treat known persistent and metastatic disease; this application will be discussed later.

The European Association of Nuclear Medicine advocates thyroid ablation in all patients, except in those with a very low risk of surgical failure—i.e. papillary carcinoma <1 cm in diameter. However, in case of a history of external irradiation, unfavourable histopathology or infiltration beyond the thyroid capsule, and even patients with tumours <1 cm ablation should be the treatment of choice. Other guidelines are more cautious. According to the European Consensus, only patients with large tumours (T3/T4) or lymph node metastases require radioiodine treatment. However, the decision to treat patients with tumours of 1–4 cm, without lymph node metastases, is left to the discretion of the treating physician, because there is no clear consensus on radioiodine treatment for this group of patients.

A number of large, retrospective studies supporting the use of radioiodine as adjuvant therapy have shown a significant reduction in the rates of recurrence. A large, pooled analysis showed a statistically significant treatment effect of ablation for the following 10-year outcomes: loco-regional recurrence (relative risk of 0.31, 95 % CI 0.2–0.49) and distant metastases (absolute decrease in risk 3 %; 95 % CI, risk 1 –4 %). Studies have also reported increased cancer-specific survival if postoperative radioiodine treatment is applied.

Success of radioiodine treatment depends to a great extent on previous surgical treatment. The larger the thyroid remnant, the lower the rate of its successful ablation. Thyroid remnants that are <2 g are considered to be 'small' and amenable to radioiodine treatment. This information comes from a meta-analysis by Doi and Woodhouse, which found the size of the thyroid remnant to be an important determinant predicting the need for total thyroid ablation with ^{131}I. Another study by Maxon et al. found that 94 % of patients had successful ablation when the surgeon left <2 g of thyroid tissue compared with a 68 % success rate when the remnant was larger. Although treatment of large thyroid remnants is not recommended routinely, it should be considered in patients with a high risk of morbidity during completion thyroidectomy.

Radioiodine Treatment of Distant Metastases

Although radioiodine uptake is ~10 times lower in cancer cells than in normal thyrocytes, in most cases it is sufficient for successful palliative or even radical treatment (Fig. 13.1). In case of metastatic disease, ^{131}I activities are higher and range from 100 to 200 mCi (3.7–7.4 GBq). Treatments are usually repeated every 6–12 months. In the group of patients with radioiodine-avid lung metastases, a 10-year survival of 84 % can be achieved. The best therapeutic effect—partial or complete remission—is observed during the first cycles of therapy, usually before the total accumulated activity exceeds 500 mCi (18.5 GBq).

In approximately one-third of patients, distant metastases are non-functional and do not concentrate radioiodine. The studies attempting redifferentiation with retinoic acid, for inducing or increasing radioiodine uptake, were not successful. Some of these patients may benefit from local treatment modalities (surgery, external

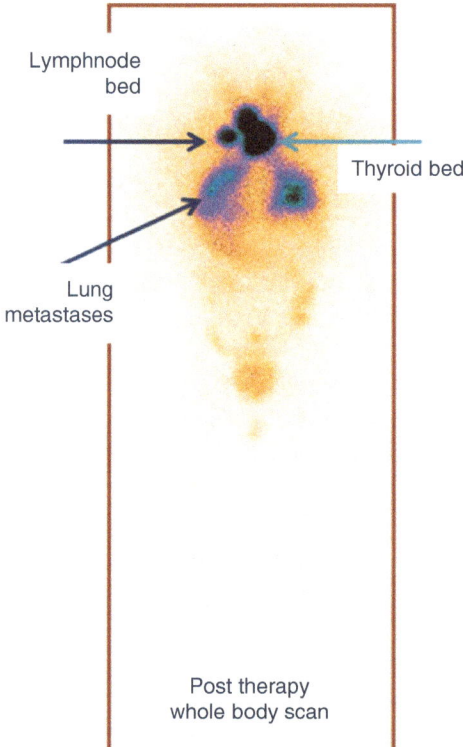
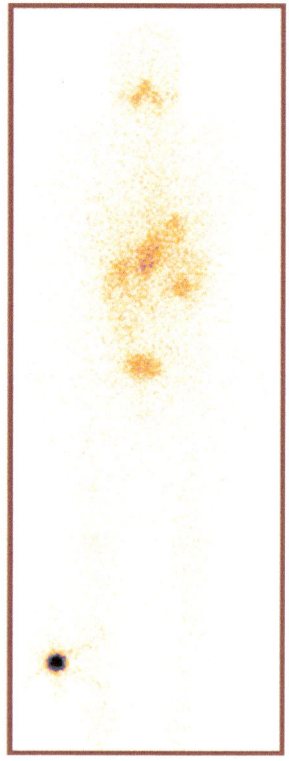

Fig. 13.1 Successful radioiodine treatment of lung and lymph node metastases of a 15-year-old female. Lung metastases were visible only on radioiodine scintigraphy (computed tomography of lung was normal). The girl was treated with 14.5 GBq (392 mCi) of ^{131}I under endogenous TSH stimulation. During the last ^{131}I treatment there was only faint uptake in the mediastinum. Stimulated thyroglobulin decreased from 1667 to 1.7 ng/ml. Six years after the diagnosis of disseminated DTC follow-up dxWBS was normal and stimulated Tg was 0.26 ng/ml (Tg antibodies absent)

beam radiotherapy, radiofrequency or [chemo] embolization). However, in the absence of effective standard treatment, these patients are good candidates for a clinical trial on new drugs, e.g. kinase inhibitors.

Patient Preparation for Radioiodine Treatment

To optimize ^{131}I uptake, radioiodine must be administered during TSH stimulation. There are two ways to do this, viz. deprive the patient of thyroid hormone or inject the patient with thyrotrophin alfa (recombinant human TSH, rhTSH).

Traditionally, TSH stimulation has been achieved after withdrawing L-T4 for 4–6 weeks, after which TSH levels are expected to be above an arbitrary cut-off of 25–30 mU/L; otherwise, withdrawal should be prolonged for another 1–2 weeks. To decrease the duration of symptoms of hypothyroidism, one can start triiodthyronine (T3) on the day L-T4 was stopped. The T3 is taken for 2–4 weeks and stopped 2 weeks before ^{131}I therapy.

Recombinant human TSH (Thyrogen™, Genzyme, Cambridge, MA) is a new but already well accepted alternative to thyroid hormone withdrawal, approved for thyroid remnant ablation in adult patients and for diagnostic studies (radioiodine scanning and Tg testing). It is given as a 0.9 mg i.m. injection on two consecutive days, causing serum TSH levels to rise immediately and to peak at ~48 h after the first injection, falling to normal levels within ~4–6 days (Fig. 13.2). Approximately 10 % of patients report side-effects, most commonly symptoms of asthaenia (the loss of strength and energy), mild headache and/or nausea. The symptoms can increase in painful bone metastases. A prospective randomized study found that thyroid hormone withdrawal and rhTSH stimulation were equally effective in preparing patients for ^{131}I remnant ablation with 100 mCi (3.7 GBq), with significantly improved quality of life. In addition, short-term recurrence rates have been found to be similar in patients prepared with thyroid hormone withdrawal or rhTSH.

To further optimize radioiodine uptake in residual thyroid cancer microfoci, it is claimed that a low-iodine diet should be started 1–2 weeks before therapy. Daily iodine intake can be decreased by restricting the use of dairy products, seafood, corned foods and salt. The application of rhTSH for radioidine treatment has raised concern about its decreased activity because of the iodine content of L-T4 preparations. Yet, a recent study indicates that the body iodine content is not an important determinant of thyroid ablation when preparing the patients with either thyroid hormone withdrawal or rhTSH.

Remnant ablation can be achieved by either administering an empirical fixed activity of ^{131}I or by using dosimetry-guided techniques. However, because of technical and logistic problems, most centres have adapted the fixed-dose or standard-dose technique for ^{131}I remnant ablation with activities ranging from 30 to 100 mCi (1.1–3.7 GBq). Multiple studies have compared the efficacy of various amounts of ^{131}I given to ablate a thyroid remnant, with a successful rate ranging from ~80 to ~100 %. A pooled analysis by Hackshaw et al., which compared the efficacy of remnant ablation following low activity (~30 mCi) versus high activity (~100 mCi) of ^{131}I, found that the average success rate of low activity was 10 % lower using

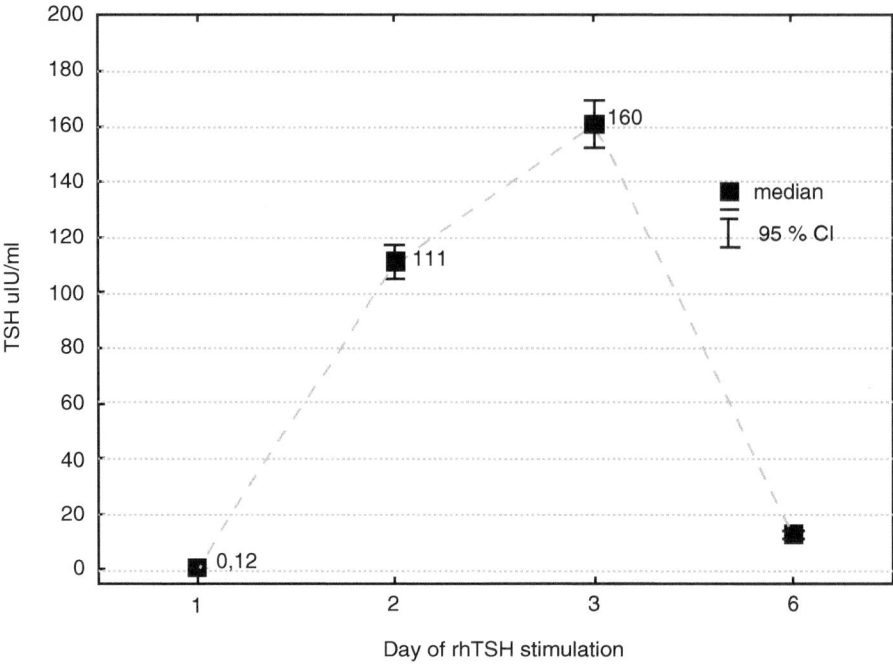

Fig. 13.2 Changes in TSH level after rhTSH stimulation. Own data based on 214 rhTSH-aided radioiodine therapies in 43 patients with disseminated thyroid cancer

30 mCi compared with 100 mCi (95 % CI 3 –17 %). In the meta analysis of Doi and Woodhouse, the difference was even larger – 77 % versus 53 % success rate for high and low activities. However, when Hackshaw et al. performed a meta-analysis of only randomized trials, no difference in success rate was seen between low and high activity. So, at present the problem of the best ^{131}I activity is still unresolved, especially in low-risk DTC patients. In patients with a high risk of persistent disease or recurrence, ^{131}I activity of 100 mCi (3.7 GBq) is recommended.

Radioiodine treatment is well tolerated. The potential, transient side-effects are mild and include nausea, taste disturbance, salivary swelling and menstrual/male reproductive tract disturbances. Dry mouth, early menopause and increased risk of secondary cancers are rare late complications. The risk of most complications increases with the cumulated radioiodine activity. Thus, it becomes more essential in the treatment of functional metastases.

Thyroid Hormone Replacement Therapy

It is generally agreed that all thyroid cancer patients must be treated post-thyroidectomy with thyroid hormones to correct surgically induced hypothyroidism and to suppress the ability of TSH to act as a growth factor for DTC.

TSH stimulates both the growth and functional activity of thyroid follicular cells. Thyrocytes' growth is promoted directly by TSH binding to its receptor (TSH-R) and also indirectly, by stimulating the secretion of autocrine growth factors and amyloid precursors, or the expression of growth factor receptors, e.g. epithelial growth factor. Most, but not all, DTCs express TSH-R. However, post-translational modification, especially by glycosylation and correct protein folding, mainly determines its functional status.

Clinical studies have demonstrated that TSH is correlated with the clinical course of thyroid cancer. Dunhill et al. were the first to observe a regression of PTC in two patients treated with thyroid hormone. Since then, cases of lymph node or distant metastases and an increase in size during prolonged periods of thyroid hormone withdrawal or rhTSH stimulation have been reported; shrinkage was found after thyroid hormone therapy. Furthermore, thyroid hormone treatment has been found to reduce the recurrence rate and cancer-related mortality in clinical studies. A large meta-analysis has suggested an association between thyroid hormone suppression therapy and reduction of major adverse clinical events.

Clear information on the optimal TSH level in patients with DTC is lacking. However, it is agreed unequivocally that TSH should be suppressed in high-risk patients or patients with persistent/recurrent disease. The appropriate degree of TSH suppression by L-T4 is still unknown. No prospective studies have been performed to examine the risk of recurrence and death from thyroid cancer associated with varying serum TSH levels. However, results of a few recent, retrospective studies are available. In two studies, constantly suppressed TSH below 0.05 or 0.1 mU/L showed a beneficial effect, especially in high-risk patients. Two other studies found that either there was no effect of TSH suppression or that a serum TSH threshold of 2 mU/L differentiated best between patients free of disease and those with relapse or cancer-related mortality.

Together, these studies indicate that in patients with a persistent or high risk of recurrence, TSH level should be suppressed, preferably below 0.1 mU/L. On the other hand, in very low-risk patients (papillary microcarcinoma) it can be kept within the lower normal range. In patients with an intermediate risk of recurrence, who are clinically and biochemically free of disease, the TSH level may be kept just below the normal range, i.e. 0.1–0.4 mU/L, or if TSH suppression is contraindicated, within the low–normal range. After 5–10 years of uneventful follow up, all patients, except those with persistent disease, may have a TSH level within the lower normal range.

The L-T4 dose required to suppress TSH is roughly correlated with the patient's weight and age. Younger patients, especially children, require higher doses per kg of body weight. In adult patients, the L-T4 dose is usually between 1.2 and 2.4 μg/kg body weight, whereas in a child it can be as high as 3–4 μg/kg. As L-T4 has a blood half-life of 6–8 days, a single daily dose is sufficient. After oral administration, ≤80 % of L-T4 is absorbed from the gut, given the inter-individual variability. Food intake is an important factor that reduces L-T4 absorption; patients should be informed that they should ingest their L-T4 dose on an empty stomach, preferably early in the morning, 30–60 min before breakfast. Some substances are known to interfere with L-T4 absorption in the gut (calcium carbonate, ferrous sulphate, soy preparations and high-fibre intake). In addition, several chronic diseases, such as achlorhydria, gastritis, regional enteritis and pancreatic diseases may be associated with decreased L-T4 absorption.

The effectiveness of L-T4 therapy is controlled by serum TSH measurement with ultra-sensitive assays 2–3 months after the therapy has been introduced. The daily dose of L-T4 has to be increased or decreased (usually by 25 µg) in the case of either too high or too low a level of TSH.

The issue of side-effects of L-T4 therapy on the target organs (mainly heart and bone) in patients requiring long-term suppressive L-T4 therapy is still controversial. Some studies have indicated that L-T4 suppressive therapy may be associated with variable degrees of bone loss, thus early prevention of osteoporosis should be considered. Long-term TSH suppression has been associated with an increased nocturnal and daytime heart rate, frequent premature arterial beats, increased left ventricular regular mass index, and systolic function. To decrease the risk of L-T4-related side-effects, serum T3 during L-T4 therapy should be kept within the normal range.

External Beam Radiation Therapy in Differentiated Thyroid Cancer

External beam radiotherapy (RT) is not clearly indicated in the management of PTC, except for palliation of inoperable local disease or distant metastases.

Patients with a gross residual tumour after attempted surgical resection, or with an inoperable tumour, are unlikely to benefit from ^{131}I radiation treatment as a single treatment unless a highly absorbed radiation dose is achieved. Hence, radioiodine treatment combined with external radiation increases the likelihood of long-term palliation. Patients in a large study ($n = 124$) with gross residual loco-regional disease after surgery for PTC were stratified according to whether or not they received RT post-surgery Patients who received RT had a significantly greater loco-regional control rate at 5-year follow up (67 % versus 38 %; p=0.001). Other retrospective studies have reported a disease control rate of 45–65 %. RT is also highly effective in palliation of bone pain or airway obstruction caused by neoplastic infiltration.

Patients with minimal extrathyroid extension or with only lymph metastases probably do not benefit from external beam RT. In a retrospective study mentioned earlier, patients >60 years of age with minimal extrathyroid extension and RT had a worse cause-specific mortality (81 % versus 65 %) and loco-regional relapse-free rate (86 % versus 65 %) than patients without RT. The Multicentre Study on Differentiated Thyroid Cancer planned as a prospective multicentre trial on the benefit of adjuvant RT in locally invasive DTC (pT4; *see* Chap. 5) failed because of poor enrolment, and after a 3-year trial became a prospective, observational cohort study. The trial showed a weak benefit of external beam RT in terms of local control, however, without statistical significance.

Chemotherapy in Differentiated Thyroid Cancer

Historically the effectiveness of systemic therapy for advanced metastatic thyroid carcinoma has been poor, with a typical response rate of ≤25 %. Because of the poor outcome, patients have been treated with cytotoxic drugs only when they become symptomatic or the cancer becomes rapidly progressive. Doxorubicin was administered most frequently on the basis of a small, uncontrolled study that reported surprisingly high, but short-lived, responses.

The recent advent of targeted therapy is a promising modality in the treatment of advanced malignancies, including DTC. The term 'targeted therapy' refers to a new generation of cancer drugs designed to interfere with a specific molecular target, typically a protein that is believed to have a critical role in tumour growth or progression. Therefore, the objective of this therapy, in contrast to standard chemotherapy, is to disrupt pathways that are inappropriately activated in cancer cells rather than directly kill malignant cells. Of prime importance in the development of targeted therapies has been the discovery of key aetiological, oncogenic mutations in PTC. The main oncogenic alteration, seen in ~80 % of PTC, is the activation of the mitogen-activated protein kinase (MAPK) pathway that leads to cell growth and proliferation. Several multikinase inhibitors have already been tested in clinical trials with DTC; they inhibit oncogenic kinases at the MAPK pathway—*BRAF* or *RET*—and simultaneously, multiple growth factor receptors. Anti-VEGFR (vascular endothelial growth factor receptor) influence is the most important for the anti-angiogenesis effect of multikinase inhibitors, which constitutes a strong, if not most important, part of their action (reviewed in Sherman 2009). Other novel approaches of potential significance are also in practice. As cytotoxic chemotherapy is of little benefit in advanced DTC, the most reasonable approach towards these patients is to enrol them in clinical trials of novel anticancer drugs.

Long-Term Follow-Up Strategy in Differentiated Thyroid Cancer After Initial Treatment

After the initial therapy, the objective of follow up is to maintain adequate TSH levels with L-T4 therapy (and in case of postoperative hypoparathyroidism, supplementation with calcium and vitamin D3 derivatives) and to detect recurrent disease. Long-term follow up is necessary because DTC can recur at any time after initial treatment and treatment with L-T4 is lifelong.

Although the protocol for follow up of patients with DTC will differ from centre to centre, three investigations play an essential role—neck ultrasound, serum Tg concentration, and ^{131}I whole-body diagnostic scintigraphy (dxWBS). Their use in follow-up protocols should be adapted to the risk of recurrence.

Neck Ultrasound

It is well known that the most frequent site of PTC recurrence is lymph nodes in the neck. Neck ultrasound with a high-frequency linear probe (>7.5 MHz) can detect lymph node metastases as small as a few millimetres. Lymph nodes are suspicious when they are hypoechogenic, lack an echogenic hilum, have a round shape, and/or have a hypervascularized appearance on colour Doppler. Microcalcifications or a cystic component is highly suspicious. The sensitivity of neck ultrasound for detecting lymph node metastases was shown to range from 97 to 100 % when combined with serum Tg measurements following TSH stimulation (*see also* Chap. 4).

Serum Thyroglobulin

Serum Tg measurements play a central role in the follow up of patients with thyroid cancer. Although this method is clearly the most sensitive means of detecting persistent or recurrent disease, it is not without its limitations. First, if thyroid remnants are present, it is not possible to differentiate whether the source of Tg is normal or neoplastic tissue. Second, because the maturation and secretion of a mature Tg molecule is complex, circulating Tg is heterogeneous, and when tumours dedifferentiate they can lose their capability to synthesize, iodinate or, more rarely, secrete conformationally normal Tg protein. Consequently, current Tg immunometric assays, based on monoclonal antibodies with restricted epitope specificity, may only recognize a limited population of Tg isoforms secreted by a neoplasm. This causes method-to-method variability in results and precludes changing assays when serially monitoring DTC patients. Third, interference with Tg antibodies (TgAb) and heterophilic antibodies can lead to the reporting of falsely low or high serum Tg values, respectively. All sera sent for Tg measurement require adjunctive TgAb testing, because the TgAb status of the patient can change over time from positive to negative and vice versa.

After resection of thyroid cancer, Tg falls with a half-life of 3–4 days. Apart from Tg released secondary to operation trauma, the dominant influences on postoperative serum Tg concentrations are the mass of remaining thyroid tissue (normal remnant and any tumour) together with the prevailing TSH status. Serum Tg reaches its nadir approximately a month after surgery.

In the absence of antibody interference, serum Tg has a high degree of sensitivity and specificity for detecting thyroid cancer. Thyroglobulin can be measured either during L-T4 suppressive therapy or after TSH stimulation, with a higher sensitivity noted following the latter. TSH stimulation encompasses either thyroid hormone withdrawal or stimulation using rhTSH (becoming increasingly popular). However, in the latter case, Tg response is typically almost twofold lower than that which occurs after L-T4 withdrawal. It is now well accepted that in patients who have undergone total or near-total thyroidectomy with ^{131}I remnant ablation, suppressed Tg level should be undetectable, i.e. defined as a serum Tg level of <1 ng/ml. However, ~20 % of patients with undetectable, suppressed Tg will show a rise to >2 ng/ml after TSH stimulation, and >36 % of these patients will harbour metastases. Currently, there is an agreement that a Tg cut-off level of >2 ng/ml after rhTSH stimulation is highly sensitive in identifying patients with a persistent tumour; it should be used in clinical practice to identify patients in need of additional diagnostic procedures.

That serum Tg measurements may fail to identify patients with residual tumour or early recurrence in the cervical lymph nodes is well proven. For this reason the best way to diagnose neck recurrence is to combine serum Tg measurements with neck ultrasound.

Radioiodine Whole-Body Scan

dxWBS has been used for many years to follow up patients with DTC. It can be performed either after thyroid hormone withdrawal or after recombinant TSH administration and, again, the latter may be recommended for avoiding hypothyroidism. The scan is conducted 48–72 h after administration of 2–5 mCi (74–185 MBq) [131]I.

There is much discussion on the need for diagnostic dxWBS in the follow up of low-risk patients with or without thyroid remnant ablation. The rationale for avoiding dxWBS at the examination performed after the first 6–12-months for patients with no evidence of disease on biochemical and neck ultrasound examinations is twofold. First, ablation (defined as the absence of uptake or a low but not measurable uptake in the thyroid bed) at a dxWBS performed after adjuvant radioiodine treatment is achieved in almost all patients who have undergone total or near-total thyroidectomy. Second, recent studies with L-T4 withdrawal or rhTSH have shown that in this setting no patient who was Tg-negative (defined as having a value below the limits of detectability) was dxWBS-positive (defined as having uptake outside the thyroid bed).

Nevertheless, this modality is still of great importance in patients with an elevated, stimulated Tg level. Data showed that 76 % of patients in whom stimulated Tg rose to >2 ng/ml had residual disease on rTSH scan. Nevertheless, the same was true for 13 % of those whose stimulated Tg level was ≤2 ng/ml. Therefore, although stimulated Tg alone may be sufficient in low-risk patients, the addition of dxWBS is essential for monitoring a high-risk population.

In patients with persisting Tg antibodies, in whom neck ultrasound is the main method of monitoring, it is necessary to perform a periodic ^{131}I scan, as serum Tg determination is not reliable in excluding persistent disease.

Follow Up of Patients with Elevated Serum Thyroglobulin but Negative Radioiodine Scintigraphy and Neck Ultrasound

Patients with detectable Tg but negative whole-body scan and no signs of recurrence on conventional imaging represent one of the most challenging issues in the management of thyroid cancer. High ^{131}I activity was found to increase the sensitivity of the whole-body scan, with visualization of neoplastic foci not seen with diagnostic scans. However, this was not confirmed in all studies.

Dedifferentiated, progressive thyroid cancer lesions that have lost their ability to concentrate radioiodine often exhibit increased metabolic activity, as reflected in enhanced glucose utilization. They can thus be detected by ^{18}F-fluorodeoxyglucose (FDG), using positron-emission tomography (PET), by which metastatic disease can be found in 50–70 % of patients. The optimal conditions to perform FDG-PET in DTC are still not well established. Nevertheless, recent studies indicate that [18]FDG-PET scans during L-T4 therapy detect fewer metastatic lesions, but the sensitivity per patient is similar to [18]FDG-PET during TSH stimulation.

The detection rate of [18]FDG-PET may depend on the Tg level. In a study by Schluter et al., positive [18]FDG-PET scan results were achieved in 11 % of patients with Tg levels of ≤10 ng/ml; this increased to 50 % in patients with Tg levels between 10 and 20 ng/ml, and to 93 % at Tg levels of >100 ng/ml. Thus, only patients with a serum Tg level of ≥10 ng/ml should be considered for a [18]FDG-PET scan.

Follow-Up Schedule in DTC Patients

Serum Tg measurement and neck ultrasound are the mainstay of follow up in patients with DTC.

- Approximately 3 months after the initial treatment has finished, serum Tg (with TgAb) and TSH should be measured.
- The complex evaluation is performed 6–12 months after the initial treatment and should consist of stimulated Tg and ^{131}I whole-body scan, depending on risk factors. Patients with a Tg of <2 ng/ml without other signs of persistent or recurrent disease can be followed with continued L-T4 therapy alone, reserving additional therapies for those patients with serum Tg levels that are rising over time, or with other evidence of disease progression (Fig. 13.3). If stimulated Tg is >2 ng/ml, imaging techniques should be employed to localize the source of Tg.
- Metastatic disease necessitates treatment tailored to the functional status of the disease.

Conclusion

Postoperative management of DTC is challenging in view of the fact that data from prospective randomized trials is scant. The therapeutic approach is based mostly on large retrospective studies, expert opinions and empirical experience. For this reason, postoperative treatment differs among centres. Still, the following points for the management of patients are accepted universally:

- Postoperative treatment and follow up should always be adjusted to the patient's risk stratification.
- All high-risk patients should be treated with radioiodine.
- Patients with papillary microcarcinoma should not be submitted to this kind of therapy unless additional risk factors are diagnosed.

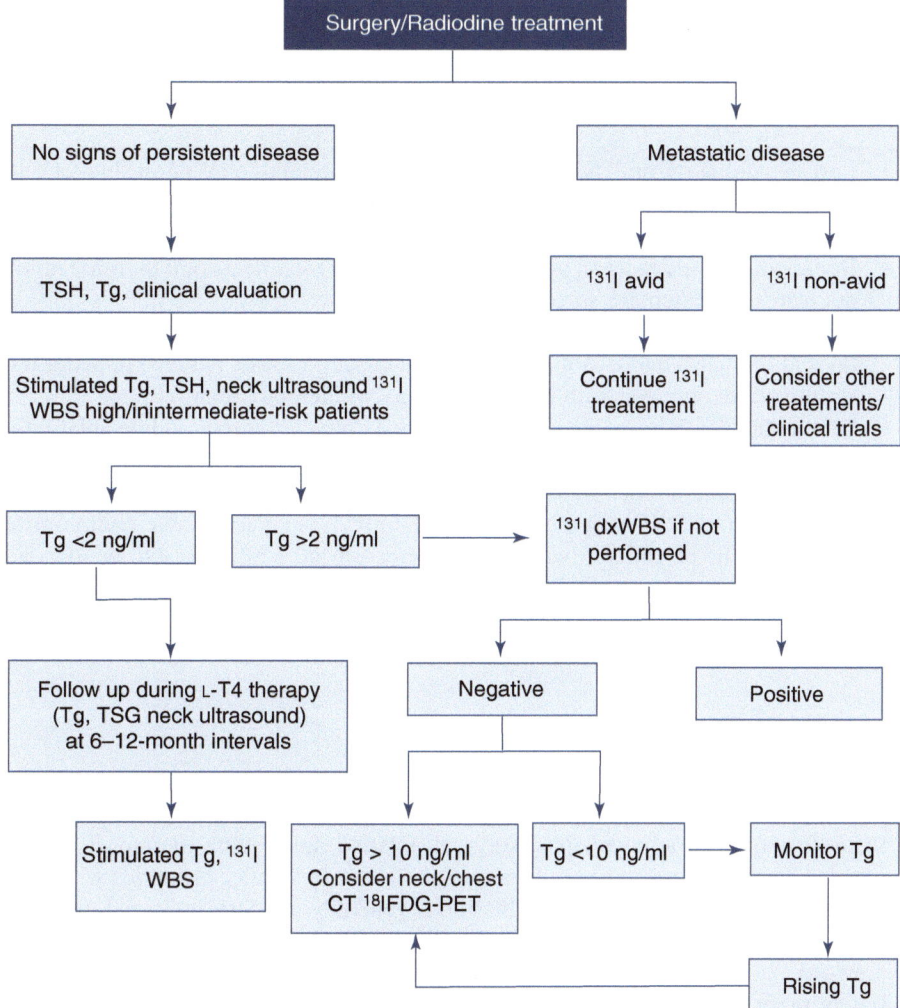

Fig. 13.3 Follow up of patients after total/near-total thyreoidectomy and radioiodine treatment

- All DTC patients need L-T4 therapy post-surgery. However, the degree of TSH suppression depends on cancer risk. Only in patients with persistent/progressive DTC is steady suppression of TSH <0.1 mU/l recommended unquestionably.
- Neck ultrasound and serum Tg should be the mainstay of DTC follow up, unless recurrent/persistent disease is suspected; in that case, other diagnostic modalities should be included.

Common Mistakes

The following points are sometimes misunderstood and should be considered during planning and performing adjuvant DTC treatment:

- Post-thyroid surgery: The volume of thyroid remnants may be evaluated with sonography only when postoperative oedema subsides (usually not before 1–2 months).
- Radioiodine is given as an adjuvant treatment for total/near-total thyroidectomy, not instead of extensive surgery.
- The clinical benefit of adjuvant radioiodine therapy lies not only in ablation of thyroid remnants and treatment of residual cancer disease, but also in better risk stratification, obtained with the post-therapy whole-body scan.
- Faint uptake of radioiodine in the thyroid bed, found after radioiodine ablation of thyroid remnants, is not an indication for repeated radioiodine if stimulated Tg is not increased and other signs of persistent disease is absent.
- Suppression of TSH with a goal of 0.1–0.4 mU/L is an acceptable compromise, which may be considered when full suppression <0.1 mU/L has to be avoided, but higher risk assessment does not permit lowering the L-T4 dose to substitutive levels.

Commentary

Markus Luster

In most countries, adjuvant post-surgical ablative radioiodine therapy is recommended for DTC with tumour diameters of >1 cm. In smaller primaries with a so-called 'very low-risk profile', ^{131}I ablation is generally not performed and may only be beneficial in the following special settings: familial history of thyroid cancer, previous external beam radiation to the neck and unfavourable histological variants. Lately, there has been some debate on whether 'low-risk' patients should receive ^{131}I ablation after total thyroidectomy. The issue of whether adjuvant radioiodine treatment is beneficial and, if so, in which patients, is a nearly irresolvable issue unless a randomized, controlled trial is conducted. In a recent study, Verburg et al. were able to show that after successful ablation, 'high-risk' patients have a recurrence-free and tumour-specific survival that does not differ from patients who were initially classified as 'low risk'. Consequently, after successful ablation the follow-up protocols in low-risk and high-risk patients need not differ. The benefits and potential risks for patients undergoing radioiodine therapy for treatment of thyroid cancer, however, must be evaluated carefully.

In most centres, standard fixed activities of 1–3 GBq are commonly used for ^{131}I ablation. The amount of activity that should be administered is still a matter of debate; randomized trials that are currently under way in Great Britain and France might answer this question. Some approaches also use a patient-specific tailoring of the activity on the basis of the radiation-absorbed dose to the blood or the target dose to the lesion(s). The main disadvantage in using a fixed-activity approach is the failure to consider the individuality of the patient. The 'optimal' activity of radioiodine to treat thyroid carcinoma is the lowest possible amount of radioiodine that delivers a lethal dose of radiation to the entire lesion/metastasis, while minimizing side-effects. Recently, [124]I (half-life 4.2 days) PET has been introduced by some groups with a special interest in pre-therapeutic dosimetry.

Empirical fixed activities, by their very nature, make no attempt to determine either the minimal radioiodine activity that will deliver a lethal dose or the maximum allowable, reasonably safe absorbed dose. Patient-specific blood-based dosimetry is comparatively easy to perform before and during therapy. In selected cases, this procedure will allow extending the activity beyond the limit of therapies using fixed activities, and will reduce the risk of severe side-effects. The determinant for a successful ^{131}I ablation is the radiation dose to the target tissue; the decisive parameters for this are the administered therapeutic activity and the retention of radioiodine in the target volume. Target tissue uptake must be expected to depend on the availability of ^{131}I in the blood. Low, mean absorbed doses are associated with poor tumour responses, but even in the presence of adequate ^{131}I uptake, cure is rarely observed in patients who are older, have a large tumour burden, and/or poorly differentiated tumours, suggesting a decreased radiosensitivity. In such patients, FDG (glucose) uptake in PET/CT is usually high (the so-called 'flip-flop phenomenon'). In those cases, a multidisciplinary approach based on individual risk stratification is warranted.

Preparation for the procedure using radioactive iodine requires a low-iodine diet for some weeks and, whenever feasible, exogenous TSH stimulation using i.m. injections of recombinant human TSH. The advantages of recombinant TSH are avoidance of morbidity associated with clinical hypothyroidism and a maintained quality of life, as well as a lower radiation dose to the remainder of the body, e.g. the bone marrow.

In general, the increasing incidence and shift towards younger patients with less aggressive tumours should stimulate discussion regarding modification of established regimens or, as Tuttle postulated recently, seeking 'Proper balance between aggressive intervention and appreciation of the potential side-effects of our well meaning efforts'.

Suggested Reading

Biermann M, Pixberg M, Riemann B, *et al.* [Clinical outcomes of adjuvant external-beam radiotherapy for differentiated thyroid cancer—results after 874 patient-years of follow-up in the MSDS-trial.] *Nuklearmedizin* 2009;**48**:89–98.

Cooper DS, Doherty GM, Haugen BR, *et al.* Revised American Thyroid Association management guidelines for patients with thyroid nodules and differentiated thyroid cancer. *Thyroid* 2009;**19**:1167–214.

David A, Blotta A, Bondanelli M, *et al.* Serum thyroglobulin concentrations and ^{131}I whole-body scan results in patients with differentiated thyroid carcinoma after administration of recombinant human thyroid-stimulating hormone. *J Nucl Med* 2001;**42**:1470–5.

Doi SA, Woodhouse NJ. Ablation of the thyroid remnant and ^{131}I dose in differentiated thyroid cancer. *Clin Endocrinol (Oxf)* 2000;**52**:765–73.

Durante C, Haddy N, Baudin E, *et al.* Long-term outcome of 444 patients with distant metastases from papillary and follicular thyroid carcinoma: Benefits and limits of radioiodine therapy. *J Clin Endocrinol Metab* 2006;**91**:2892–9.

Eustatia-Rutten CF, Smit JW, Romijn JA, *et al.* Diagnostic value of serum thyroglobulin measurements in the follow-up of differentiated thyroid carcinoma, a structured meta-analysis. *Clin Endocrinol (Oxf)* 2004;**61**:61–74.

Glanzmann C, Lutolf UM. Long-term follow-up of 92 patients with locally advanced follicular or papillary thyroid cancer after combined treatment. *Strahlenther Onkol* 1992;**168**:260–9.

Gottlieb JA, Hill CS, Jr. Chemotherapy of thyroid cancer with adriamycin. Experience with 30 patients. *N Engl J Med* 1974;**290**:193–7.

Hackshaw A, Harmer C, Mallick U, *et al.* [131]I activity for remnant ablation in patients with differentiated thyroid cancer: A systematic review. *J Clin Endocrinol Metab* 2007;**92**:28–38.

Handkiewicz-Junak D, Roskosz J, Hasse-Lazar K, *et al.* 13-cis-retinoic acid re-differentiation therapy and recombinant human thyrotropin-aided radioiodine treatment of non-functional metastatic thyroid cancer: A single-center, 53-patient phase 2 study. *Thyroid Res* 2009;**2**:8.

Handkiewicz-Junak D, Wloch J, Roskosz J, *et al.* Total thyroidectomy and adjuvant radioiodine treatment independently decrease locoregional recurrence risk in childhood and adolescent differentiated thyroid *cancer. J Nucl Med* 2007;**48**:879–88.

Handkiewicz-Junak D, Czarniecka A, Jarzab B. Molecular prognostic markers in papillary and follicular thyroid cancer: Current status and future directions. *Mol Cell Endocrinol* 2010;**322**:8–28.

Haugen BR, Pacini F, Reiners C, *et al.* A comparison of recombinant human thyrotropin and thyroid hormone withdrawal for the detection of thyroid remnant or cancer. *J Clin Endocrinol Metab* 1999;**84**:3877–85.

Helal BO, Merlet P, Toubert ME, *et al.* Clinical impact of (18)F-FDG PET in thyroid carcinoma patients with elevated thyroglobulin levels and negative ^{131}I scanning results after therapy. *J Nucl Med* 2001;**42**:1464–9.

Hindie E, Melliere D, Lange F, *et al.* Functioning pulmonary metastases of thyroid cancer: Does radioiodine influence the prognosis? *Eur J Nucl Med Mol Imaging* 2003;**30**:974–81.

Hovens GC, Stokkel MP, Kievit J, *et al.* Associations of serum thyrotropin concentrations with recurrence and death in differentiated thyroid cancer. *J Clin Endocrinol Metab* 2007;**92**:2610–15.

Jonklaas J, Sarlis NJ, Litofsky D, *et al.* Outcomes of patients with differentiated thyroid carcinoma following initial therapy. *Thyroid* 2006;**16**:1229–42.

Leboulleux S, Schroeder PR, Busaidy NL, *et al.* Assessment of the incremental value of recombinant thyrotropin stimulation before 2-[18F]-Fluoro-2-deoxy-D-glucose positron emission tomography/computed tomography imaging to localize residual differentiated thyroid cancer. *J Clin Endocrinol Metab* 2009;**94**:1310–16.

Luster M, Clarke SE, Dietlein M, *et al.* Guidelines for radioiodine therapy of differentiated thyroid cancer. *Eur J Nucl Med Mol Imaging* 2008;**35**:1941–59.

Maxon HR III, Englaro EE, Thomas SR, *et al.* Radioiodine-131 therapy for well-differentiated thyroid cancer—a quantitative radiation dosimetric approach: Outcome and validation in 85 patients. *J Nucl Med* 1992;**33**:1132–6.

Mazzaferri EL, Kloos RT. Clinical review 128: Current approaches to primary therapy for papillary and follicular thyroid cancer. *J Clin Endocrinol Metab* 2001;**86**:1447–63.

Mazzaferri EL, Robbins RJ, Spencer CA, *et al.* A consensus report of the role of serum thyroglobulin as a monitoring method for low-risk patients with papillary thyroid carcinoma. *J Clin Endocrinol Metab* 2003;**88**:1433–41.

McGriff NJ, Csako G, Gourgiotis L, *et al.* Effects of thyroid hormone suppression therapy on adverse clinical outcomes in thyroid cancer. *Ann Med* 2002;**34**:554–64.

O'Connell ME, Flower MA, Hinton PJ, *et al.* Radiation dose assessment in radioiodine therapy. Dose–response relationships in differentiated thyroid carcinoma using quantitative scanning and PET. *Radiother Oncol* 1993;**28**:16–26.

Pacini F, Schlumberger M, Dralle H, *et al.* European Consensus for the management of patients with differentiated thyroid carcinoma of the follicular epithelium. *Eur J Endocrinol* 2006;**154**:787–803.

Pacini F, Molinaro E, Castagna MG, *et al.* Ablation of thyroid residues with 30 mCi ^{131}I: A comparison in thyroid cancer patients prepared with recombinant human TSH or thyroid hormone withdrawal. *J Clin Endocrinol Metab* 2002;**87**:4063–8.

Pujol P, Daures JP, Nsakala N, *et al.* Degree of thyrotropin suppression as a prognostic determinant in differentiated thyroid cancer. *J Clin Endocrinol Metab* 1996;**81**:4318–23.

Sakorafas GH, Giotakis J, Stafyla V. Papillary thyroid microcarcinoma: A surgical perspective. *Cancer Treat Rev* 2005;**31**:423–38.

Sawka AM, Thephamongkhol K, Brouwers M, *et al.* Clinical review 170: A systematic review and metaanalysis of the effectiveness of radioactive iodine remnant ablation for well-differentiated thyroid cancer. *J Clin Endocrinol Metab* 2004;**89**:3668–76.

Sherman SI. Advances in chemotherapy of differentiated epithelial and medullary thyroid cancers. *J Clin Endocrinol Metab* 2009;**94**:1493–9.

Spencer CA, Bergoglio LM, Kazarosyan M, *et al.* Clinical impact of thyroglobulin (Tg) and Tg autoantibody method differences on the management of patients with differentiated thyroid carcinomas. *J Clin Endocrinol Metab* 2005;**90**:5566–75.

Tala Jury HP, Castagna MG, Fioravanti C, *et al.* Lack of association between urinary iodine excretion and successful thyroid ablation in thyroid cancer patients. *J Clin Endocrinol Metab* 2010;**95**:230–7.

Torlontano M, Attard M, Crocetti U, *et al.* Follow-up of low risk patients with papillary thyroid cancer: Role of neck ultrasonography in detecting lymph node metastases. *J Clin Endocrinol Metab* 2004;**89**:3402–7.

Tuttle RM, Brokhin M, Omry G, *et al.* Recombinant human TSH-assisted radioactive iodine remnant ablation achieves short-term clinical recurrence rates similar to those of traditional thyroid hormone withdrawal. *J Nucl Med* 2008;**49**:764–70.

Verburg FA, Mader U, Luster M, *et al.* Histology does not influence prognosis in differentiated thyroid carcinoma when accounting for age, tumour diameter, invasive growth and metastases. *Eur J Endocrinol* 2009;**160**:619–24.

Index

© The Author(s) 2012

F.L. Greene, A.L. Komorowski (eds.), *Clinical Approach to Well-differentiated Thyroid Cancers*, Head and Neck Cancer Clinics, DOI 10.1007/978-81-322-2568-3